ATKINS
DIET PLAN 2021

A Complete Guide to Lose Weight without Exercise, Improve Your Health, and Feel Amazing. Including a 31-Day Meal Plan with Recipes and a Focus on Intermittent Fasting

© Copyright 2021 - All rights reserved.

The content contained within this book may not be reproduced, duplicated or transmitted without direct written permission from the author or the publisher.

Under no circumstances will any blame or legal responsibility be held against the publisher, or author, for any damages, reparation, or monetary loss due to the information contained within this book. Either directly or indirectly.

Legal Notice:

This book is copyright protected. This book is only for personal use. You cannot amend, distribute, sell, use, quote or paraphrase any part, or the content within this book, without the consent of the author or publisher.

Disclaimer Notice:

Please note the information contained within this document is for educational and entertainment purposes only. All effort has been executed to present accurate, up to date, and reliable, complete information. No warranties of any kind are declared or implied. Readers acknowledge that the author is not engaging in the rendering of legal, financial, medical or professional advice. The content within this book has been derived from various sources. Please consult a licensed professional before attempting any techniques outlined in this book.

By reading this document, the reader agrees that under no circumstances is the author responsible for any losses, direct or indirect, which are incurred as a result of the use of information contained within this document, including, but not limited to, errors, omissions, or inaccuracies.

Table Of Contents

Introduction   6

Chapter 1: Why Atkins Diet?   8

Chapter 2: Atkins Diet And Ketogenic Diet   14

Chapter 3: 4 Steps Of Atkins Diet   16

Chapter 4: Meal Plan Day 1-7   20

Chapter 5: Meal Plan Day 8-14   48

Chapter 6: Meal Plan Day 15-21   78

Chapter 7: Meal Plan Day 22-28 **108**

Chapter 8: Meal Plan Day 29-31 **136**

Chapter 9: Atkins Diet And Intermittent Fasting   150

Conclusion   154

Introduction

More than likely, you've purchased this book because you want to learn more about the Atkins Diet; a diet that has been one of the primary health crazes over the past couple of decades, and how it can help you lose weight. Maybe you've had a health scare or you have simply got tired of looking at yourself in the mirror and wishing you were a few pounds lighter. On the other hand, maybe you don't need to lose weight and you are simply looking for a way to eat healthy and maintain your current weight. Whatever the reason may be, you've decided to go for the Atkins Diet.

Don't let all of that scare you away, though. The Atkins Diet can be simple to follow and can really help you lose the weight that you are ready to get rid of. Enough of that, though, let's go ahead and delve right into learning more about the Atkins Diet!

You've tried losing weight, but have failed. You hate to count calories or to feel that you have to restrict how much you eat, so you are always hungry. You are beginning to think that there is no hope for you.

Don't give up quite yet, because there is hope on the Atkins diet. Many people have found the answer to their weight loss question when they start to follow the low-carb plan advocated in the Atkins diet. Instead of counting calories, you count the net carbs that you eat. You don't have to feel deprived, and you are encouraged to eat enough food so that you feel satiated and full.

This book will describe the Atkins diet in detail, including the four phases of the diet, the foods that you can eat on each phase, and even some recipes that you can try. All your questions will be answered in this book. By the time you are finished, you will have all the information and the tools that you need to succeed on the Atkins diet. You can lose weight fast. In fact, many people report being able to lose up to 30 pounds in 30 days!

So, what are you waiting for? This book has the answers that you are looking for.

ХНАПТЕР 1:

Why Atkins diet?

The Atkins Diet suggests an extensive line-up of fruits low in glycemic such as avocado, healthy fats such as olive oil, vegetables, sufficient proteins and whole grains as one comes closer to their goals of weight loss.

Believe me you would not feel hungry and your desire for food would be greatly reduced, when you go on a diet with more of fat and extremely low in carbohydrates (ketogenic). There are four phases of this diet.

But what is the Atkins Diet? Basically, Atkins found that when you cut out most carbohydrates and sugars, but didn't restrict other foods, people lost weight. It's not about completely cutting out carbs, but includes eating only those carbs that are nutrient dense. His diet is based on the premise that people who cut carbs and sugars, but are able to eat anything else, will lose weight. And the results have shown this to be true. People who start on the Atkins Diet have lost up to 30 pounds in the first thirty days! The results bear themselves out. Be willing to cut out carbs and sugars, while not restricting anything else that you eat, and you can lose weight. The research has proven this.

How does this work? Basically, the idea behind the Atkins diet is that the body has two different options that they can use for fuel: either sugar from the foods you eat, or stored fats in the body. The body will use simple sugars and carbs first, because it is the easiest to utilize. If you stop eating sugars and carbohydrates, which are turned into sugars in the body, that only leaves one fuel source for your body, the fats that you have already stored. Because sugars aren't available, the body will start to metabolize the stored fats, especially those fats around the belly area, to fuel the body. And you lose weight. It is really that simple.

Phase one allows only 20-25 grams of net carbs per day and does not allow any type of carbohydrate-based foods, getting the net carbs you eat mostly from the vegetables in your diet. This is also often called the Induction phase, meaning that your body is being inducted into eating low carbs. This is the most restrictive phase of the diet, and can sometimes be tough on people who are not used to eating so few carbs. Of course, any change in diet can be difficult at first, but once you see the changes on your body and how quickly you will lose weight, you won't feel so deprived. Most people will stay in the induction phase for at least two weeks, but if you have a lot of weight to lose, you can stay in it for much longer.

Phase 2 can be started at least two weeks after phase 1, although most people wait until they are within 15 pounds of their goals weight. That means if you have a lot to lose, you won't move to phase 2 for a long time. Some people do choose to move to phase 2 earlier, but the weight will come off more slowly. You will still see weight loss, however. Phase 2 allows 25-50 grams of net carbs per day, and adds foods such as whole grains and high carb fruits. In Phase 3, you are allowed to eat from 50-80 grams of net carbs. You can start this phase when you are within 5 pounds of your goal weight.

Phase 4 is also called the lifetime maintenance phase, which is where you can go from 80-100 grams of net carbs. This is the phase that you should eat at for the rest of your life to maintain your weight loss. After all, you want to find a happy medium between being able to eat foods that you enjoy and keeping weight off. Atkins will help you progress between very restricted net carbs to finding a balance for your body to have healthy carbs added while still maintaining your weight loss.

Benefits of Following Atkins

Low-carb diets were also shown to improve the problem of daytime sleepiness in people who suffer from narcolepsy, a disorder where people uncontrollably fall asleep during the day.

As you can see, there are many benefits in following the Atkins diet. If you suffer from any of these diseases, besides losing weight, you could see some significant improvements in a variety of medical disorders!

You Will Lose Weight by Following the Atkins Diet

If you eat fewer carbs and stay at a calorie deficit, then you are going to lose weight, guaranteed! Some followers have seen drops of more than 100 pounds! The amount of weight you lose will depend on your adherence to the plan. But one thing is an absolute guarantee; if you restrict carbs, you will lose weight.

It Will Improve the Health of Your Heart

We all know that obesity significantly increases your risk of heart disease, so lowering weight will positively affect the health of your heart. Furthermore, following a low-carb diet also reduces the risk of high blood pressure. When we consume carbs, our body will produce insulin that will hold onto excess fat for later use. Low-carb dieting will decrease the bad cholesterol while boosting the good cholesterol, effectively reducing blood pressure.

Atkins is Amazing at Controlling your Appetite

At first, you might have some cravings. This will be especially true during the introduction to the Atkins diet. When you eliminate carbs, your body will start to go through carb withdrawal. You will crave sweets and sugars, but it does not take much time for your body to adapt. Once it does, your cravings will be eliminated, and you will start to experience a suppressed appetite.

Experience an Improvement in Brain Function

One of the myths surrounding low-carb diets is that they will affect your brain function in a negative way. But the truth is that once your body has adapted to the lack of carbs, then the new metabolic process of using fat as the primary fuel source will actually lead to an improvement in brain function. Healthy fats and vitamin B are both essential to improved brain function, and they are both found in foods that we'll focus on in the Atkins diet.

Improves Physical Endurance

We know that the Atkins diet can help you lose weight, but when your body starts learning to metabolize fat, you will experience a boost in performance as well. That's because burning fat is like giving your body high octane fuel to burn. The metabolic increase that you'll experience is so significant that you will be able to push yourself further.

Atkins Diet Promotes More Nutrients

By focusing on the foods that are allowed on the Atkins diet, you will be eating more nutrients than you're probably used to. These vitamins and minerals will impact your health in ways that you can't even imagine. You'll feel so much better and have much more energy to tackle your everyday life. When you eat a healthy meal, you will feel amazing afterwards, whereas when you eat meals like pizza, you feel bloated and tired afterwards.

Atkins Dieting Targets Abdominal Fat

Belly fat is one of the most dangerous types of fat because it impacts almost every organ in your body. It also produces the most harmful chemicals and hormones. Belly fat is shown to increase the risk of diabetes and cancer.

Low-carb dieting will target this fat first and you'll see it start to quickly fade. This is usually the most difficult fat to shed, but the Atkins diet will give you results that you can start to see within just a few weeks!

The Side Effects When Starting the Atkins Diet and How to Cure Them

Headache, nausea, brain fog and irritability

All these are called induction flu because they mimic the symptoms of a real flu. It mostly happens during the first four days of the diet, usually day 2 to day 4. Headache is usually the most common. The main cause is usually dehydration and/or a deficiency of salt caused by a temporary increase in urination. These symptoms disappear by themselves within a few days. The good news is that, the symptoms can often be avoided.

Bad Breath

This is not common to all, but you could be one of those who experience a characteristic smell; fruit smell that often smells like nail polish. The smell is from a ketone body called acetone. This is a sign that your body is now using ketones as the primary source of energy instead of glucose. The smell is temporary and always goes away after a week or two.

Heart Palpitations

This is common during the first few weeks. It is also common for the heart to beat harder. The main cause again is dehydration. A reduction in the amount of fluid flowing in your bloodstream means that your body will have to pump a bit harder to keep up the blood pressure. Sometimes, the palpitations are linked to stress hormones produced to maintain the blood sugar levels. This problem is temporary and should go away after a week or two.

Reduced physical performance

For a few weeks, you will realize that you don't have the energy you used to have while on a high carb diet, therefore lowering your physical performance. It takes time for your body to adapt to burning fats instead glucose. Dehydration is also another reason why you don't perform as before.

How to Follow Atkins Diet When Eating Out

With Atkins diet, you can eat at nearly any restaurant and still stick to your goal. But before you go eating out, you need to know some things about the restaurants:

Don't trust their menu. A meal could be labeled 'low-carb' or 'healthy' but it does not mean it is. Although some restaurants might have done their homework right, don't take any chances of the carb amounts not listed.

All restaurants love to keep their customers coming. Don't think twice when asking what is in your dish even if you are a regular customer. Don't assume that they know. Be specific about any changes you would like such as sauces, and salad dressings if any.

Play it safe with the salad. Be sure to order dressings that have an oil-and-vinegar base.

Exercise portion control. Some restaurants offer supersized portions to keep customers coming back. You can always take leftovers home for your dog.

Preview the menu. Today, restaurants post their menu online. Review the menu before heading to the restaurant so that you can decide what you can order. This will also save you the temptation to order dishes that are less suitable.

If you are concerned that eating in a Mexican restaurant could tempt you with a long list of high-carbohydrates favorites, then it will be best for you to go somewhere else.

For whom is the Atkins diet suitable?

For healthy, adult people, this diet is suitable.

If you suffer from kidney or liver damage, you should rather do without such a protein diet.

Even for children or young people who are still growing, the diet is not recommended because many nutrients are needed, which are important for development.

For diabetics, however, it is a good alternative, since, in the diet, very little insulin is released.

Very seriously overweight people should consult a doctor beforehand, and have their blood values checked so that a health risk can be ruled out.

Also, the Atkins diet is not for vegans or vegetarians, as the main ingredient of the diet are meat and animal products.

XHAПTEP 2:

Atkins Diet and Ketogenic Diet

They may be both low-carb diets, but the Atkins Diet and Ketogenic Diet are not exactly the same.

The most glaring difference between the two is their origins. While the Atkins Diet was primarily designed for weight management, the Ketogenic Diet (or keto diet) was originally tailored as a tool for seizure prevention as part of epilepsy treatment. It was only recently that keto diet was adopted as a strategy for losing weight.

The amount of protein intake allowed is another key difference between the Atkins Diet and keto diet. The Atkins Diet has been dubbed the "all bacon, all the time" plan as dieters under this approach get about 60 percent of daily calories from fat and 30 percent from protein. The keto diet, on the other hand, is more of "an avocado a day" plan with 75 to 90 percent of daily calories from fat and 6 to 20 percent from protein.

The carb limits imposed by the Atkins Diet and Keto Diet are also different, even though both diets use a very low-carb intake approach that triggers ketosis for weight loss. Atkins dieters get at least 10 percent of their daily calories from carbohydrates, while keto followers only consume 2 to 5 percent of calories from carbs per day.

The allowed amount of carbohydrates intake under the Atkins approach changes throughout its four phases, while keto's carbs limit is the same amount from start to end. While the Atkins Diet counts net carbs, keto diet takes all carbs into account. In the long run, the carbs limit tends to be higher under the Atkins Diet than keto diet.

Another key difference is the extent of triggering ketosis. Ketosis is at play mainly during the first and second phases of the Atkins Diet, while keto diet requires the body to be in ketosis all throughout the diet program. Atkins dieters are gradually reintroducing carbs to their diet as they progress, while keto followers' carbs intake is always restricted.

This approach on ketosis makes the Atkins Diet a more sustainable long-term diet plan. Reintroducing carbohydrates upon reaching and maintaining the desired weight brings the body out of ketosis. This is deemed healthier as ketosis can trigger a possibly fatal build-up of excess in ketones (a by-product of fat metabolism) in the blood called ketoacidosis.

According to dietitians, however, neither of these diets is recommended as a lifetime diet plan. If done short term, the Atkins Diet and keto diet can be safe for those without any chronic conditions. But those with heart- and kidney-related diseases or diabetes are prohibited from going through these two diets.

ХНАПТЕР 3:

4 steps of Atkins diet

Induction Phase

This is the most restrictive of all Atkins diet phases, and lasts for two weeks; it is the phase in which the body begins to enter the state of ketosis. Total carbohydrate intake is restricted to less than 20 grams net per day in phase 1, and is to be provided by the allowed vegetables. During this phase, the use of protein and fat rich sources of foods is encouraged. It is recommended that eight glasses of water be consumed daily, and moderate intake of caffeine is also allowed.

Drink enough water and liquids to avoid dehydration, including clear broth, soups and unsweetened beverages to help you maintain the electrolyte balance of the body. Try to avoid processed food items and avoid eating out. If you absolutely must eat out, be certain of the ingredients used in food preparation, and be wary of the hidden sources of carbohydrates. You may use sugar substitutes, but limit intake to 1 to 3 packets per day.

There are commercial products especially designed for Atkins, and the majority of them can be used during the induction phase. If you plan to continue phase 1 for more than two weeks, then you may want to add nuts and seeds to your meal plan. In conclusion, the best way to kickstart phase 1, is by including the foundation vegetables, proteins, fats, and cheeses.

Ongoing Weight Loss (OWL) Phase

This phase consists of incremental increases in carbohydrate intake, with about 5 grams of carbohydrate intake added on a weekly basis. Sources of carbohydrates are increased gradually, with the intention to avoid carbohydrate cravings. This phase lasts until weight is within 4.5 kg (10 pounds) of the target weight.

The Atkins Diet consists of a ladder of nine rungs of carbohydrate sources of foods, which are increased in a systematic manner. As you proceed from phase 1 to phase 2, you may start to increase your carbohydrate intake, beginning with nuts and seeds, proceeding to other sources accordingly; such as berries, cherries and melon, whole milk, Greek cheese, yogurt, ricotta cheese, cottage cheese, legumes and tomato juice. After the induction period is over, you may start adding more vegetables, nuts, seeds, cheeses, coconut milk, soy milk, and almond milk

Fine Tuning

Now that you're approaching your target weight, you can begin preparing for a lifetime of weight management and healthy eating habits in Phase 3, which is otherwise known as the Fine Tuning or Pre-maintenance Phase. This is your chance to adjust and perfect your low-carb diet and get rid of those last few excess pounds.

Net carb intake

During Phase 3, you will continue to gradually increase your net carb intake each week. This time though, you will increase your daily carb consumption in 10-gram increments until you drop those remaining 5 to 10 pounds or are losing less than a pound per week.

Evaluating your carb choices

Increasing the variety of carbs in your diet can be tricky, as the impact each food has on your body varies. Plus, how your body reacts may be different than what others experience, so you have to see for yourself what works and doesn't work for you. Go about this slowly and carefully, and keep close tabs on your weight. The plan is to observe how your body responds to the foods you reintroduce. If a particular food causes cravings, uncontrollable hunger and other symptoms that lead to weight gain, then you can eliminate it from your diet. Remember, even though your weight loss slows during Phase 3, you still should be losing weight.

The Pre-Maintenance Phase

This phase allows for a carbohydrate increase of 10 grams each week progressively with the key goal of finding the "Critical Carbohydrate Level for Maintenance". At this point, some of the forbidden carbohydrates will start to reappear in the meals gradually on a weekly basis, and you may

Food options

There aren't many diet restrictions in Phase 4, and you'll basically be eating the same group of foods that you did as you completed Phase 3. If your list includes full-fat yogurt, whole grains and fruits, watch your intake closely to make sure you don't overdo it. With fruits, for instance, you need to limit it to two servings per day. Also, don't forget to make room for protein and healthy fats, as these will help with moderating your blood sugar and ultimately managing your weight. You can also have occasional treats. Just don't overindulge.

Self-control and discipline

During the earlier phases, rules and boundaries were set to keep you on track. But in Phase 4, it's all on you. You are responsible for your own weight management. So, you need to push yourself and stay motivated, disciplined and in control. The good news is, with the way the Atkins diet is designed, you enter Phase 4 with the knowledge and skills to effectively deal with the challenges of maintaining a low-carb diet.

Weight gain

As hard as it is to reach your target weight, maintaining that weight can be even more challenging. That's why you need to take action right away if you notice that you're regaining a few pounds. The best thing you can do is to reduce your daily net carb intake by 10 grams or so until you're back to your target weight. You can begin by eliminating certain carb sources or minimizing your consumption of the following: banana, grapefruit, watermelon, potatoes, carrots, beets, edamame, lentils, chickpeas, oatmeal, bread and rice.

Which Foods Should be Eaten

Atkins Diet friendly foods include all types of fish, e. g. cod, trout, halibut, tuna, sole, flounder, salmon, herring, sardines

Shellfish are also allowed, including lobster, shrimp, mussels, squid, oysters, crab, clams, and prawns.

All types of meat are permitted, including veal, beef, mutton, chicken, lamb, quail, duck and turkey. Eggs in all styles and forms are approved items in this diet. Fried, soft-boiled, hard-boiled, omelets, poached, scrambled or any other sort of eggs are all acceptable.

All types of cheese are Atkins approved, including Swiss, feta, mozzarella, parmesan, cream cheese, gouda, cheddar, blue cheese, and more.

Many low carbohydrate vegetables are permitted in limited amounts, including bok choy, alfalfa sprouts, arugula, celery, chicory green, chives, jicama, fennel, escarole, endive, daikon, cucumber, green leaf lettuce, radishes, radicchio, peppers, parsley, mushrooms, and iceberg lettuce.

Herbs and spices may be included as desired, but they must be in their original forms with no additives. Allowed spices and herbs include tarragon, sage, rosemary, pepper, oregano, basil, cayenne pepper, cilantro, dill, garlic, and ginger.

Fats and oils on the Atkins list include butter, olive oil, mayonnaise, sesame seeds oil, walnut oil, almond oil, coconut oil, grape-seed oil, sunflower oil, safflower oil and all other vegetable oils. Foods restricted from the Atkins diet include whole grain cereals and all products containing whole grains; such as cakes, biscuits, buns, bread, pastries, pitas, fruits, fruit juices, all fruit products, milk, potatoes, sweet potatoes, beets, corn, legumes, alcoholic beverages, nuts and seeds.

Oysters and mussels should be limited to 4 ounces per day as these are comparatively higher in carbohydrate content than other seafoods. Processed meat may contain sugar, and should therefore be avoided. Add eggs to your breakfast meal on a daily basis, as these are considered a staple of the Atkins diet. Be creative with all the recipes, especially with breakfast egg recipes and try to add vegetables, like onions, peppers or mushrooms as often as possible; you may make them more fulfilling by adding your choice of cheese.

ХНАПТЕР 4:

Meal Plan Day 1-7

Day 1

Breakfast:

Black Beans Lunch Mix

Preparation time: 10 minutes
Cooking time: 20 minutes
Servings: 2
Ingredients:
- 30 ounces canned black beans
- 1 cup veggie stock
- 1 tablespoon olive oil
- 1 yellow onion, chopped
- 1 jalapeno, chopped
- 1 red bell pepper, chopped
- 2 garlic cloves, minced
- 1 teaspoon ginger, grated
- ½ teaspoon cumin, ground
- ½ teaspoon oregano, dried

Directions:
1. In a pan that fits your air fryer, mix all ingredients except the rice; toss.
2. Place the pan in your air fryer and cook at 360°F for 25 minutes.
3. Add the rice and toss again.
4. Divide into bowls, serve, and enjoy.

Nutrition: calories 200, fat 8g, fiber 4g, carbs 8g, protein 3g

Snack
Tuna Tomatoes Cream Cheese Wraps
Preparation Time: 20 minutes
Cooking Time: 15 minutes
Servings: 2
Ingredients
- 100g can tuna, drained
- 2 tsp. fresh lemon juice
- 180g light cream cheese
- 125g can tomatoes, drained
- 2 slices tortillas
- 2 tbsp. fresh chives, chopped

Directions:
1. Add the tuna in a mixing bowl.
2. Mix in the cream cheese.
3. Add the tomatoes, lemon juice, and chives.
4. Mix well and make sure everything is coated with each other.
5. Take a generous amount of the tuna mixture and spread onto the tortillas.
6. Wrap them tightly and seal using a toothpick.
7. Serve fresh with any sauce of your choice.
8. You can also cut the wraps in 3 pieces and serve.

Nutrition: calories 183, fat 8g, fiber 1g, carbs 3g, protein 9g

Lunch:
Roasted Turkey Breast
Preparation time: 10 minutes
Cooking Time: 50 minutes
Serving: 2
Ingredients:
- 3 lb. boneless turkey breast
- ¼ cup mayonnaise
- 2 tsp. poultry seasoning
- 1 tsp. salt
- ½ tsp. garlic powder
- ¼ tsp. black pepper

Directions:
1. Whisk all the ingredients, including turkey in a bowl, and coat it well.
2. Place the boneless turkey breast in the Air fryer basket.
3. Rotate the dial to select the "Air fry" mode.
4. Press the Time button and again use the dial to set the cooking time to 50 minutes.
5. Now press the Temp button and rotate the dial to set the temperature at 350°F.
6. Once preheated, place the air fryer basket in the Ninja® oven and Close its lid to bake.
7. Slice and serve.

Nutrition: calories 323, fat 11g, fiber 4g, carbs 13g, protein 17g

Dinner:
Enjoyable Shrimp Paella
Preparation time: 10 minutes
Cooking time: 35 minutes
Servings: 2
Ingredients:
- 1 lb. jumbo shrimp, peeled and deveined
- 1 cup cauliflower rice
- 4 tbsp. butter
- 1 onion, chopped
- 4 garlic cloves, minced
- 1 red pepper, chopped
- 1 cup chicken broth
- 5 tbsp. White wine
- ½ tsp. salt

Directions:
1. Press the Sauté button and add the butter to the Instant Pot.
2. Once the butter has melted, add the onions and cook until softened.
3. Add the garlic and cook for 1 minute, stirring occasionally.
4. Add the red pepper and seasonings and cook for 1 minute.
5. Add the cauliflower rice and cook for 1 minute, stirring frequently.
6. Add the chicken broth and white wine. Add the shrimp.
7. Close and seal the lid; cook at high pressure for 5 minutes.
8. Serve and enjoy!

Nutrition: calories 103, fat 4g, fiber 1g, carbs 3g, protein 22g

Day 2

Breakfast:
Beans and Quinoa Stew

Preparation time: 10 minutes
Cooking time: 15 minutes
Serving: 2
Ingredients:

- 30 oz. canned black beans, drained
- 1 cup quinoa
- 30 oz. canned tomatoes, chopped
- 2 sweet potatoes, cubed
- 1 yellow onion, chopped
- 1 green bell pepper, chopped
- 1 tbsp. chili powder
- 2 tbsp. cocoa powder

Directions:

1. Place all ingredients in a pan that fits your air fryer, and stir well.
2. Then put the pan in the air fryer and cook at 400°F for 15 minutes.
3. Divide into bowls and serve right away.

Nutrition: calories 200, fat 8g, fiber 4g, carbs 9g, protein 4g

Snack
Avocado Chicken Cream Cheese Snacks
Preparation Time: 15 minutes
Cooking Time: 15 minutes
Servings: 1
Ingredients:
- 1 Avocado
- 6 lavash crackers
- 1 carrot
- 1 tbsp. cream cheese
- 20g leftover chicken

Directions:
1. Peel the avocado and the carrots. Discard the seed of the avocado.
2. Scoop out the flesh of the avocado and add to a bowl.
3. Grate the carrot and add to the bowl.
4. Take one cracker and spread some cream cheese.
5. Add the carrot mix followed by the chicken.
6. Repeat with the rest of the crackers and dig in.

Nutrition: calories 110, fat 10g, fiber 1g, carbs 3g, protein 6g

Lunch:

Brine Soaked Turkey

Preparation time: 10 minutes
Cooking time: 40 minutes
Servings: 2
Ingredients:

- 7 lb. bone-in, skin-on turkey breast

Brine:

- 1/2 cup salt
- 1 lemon
- 1/2 onion
- 3 cloves garlic, smashed

Turkey Breast:

- 4 tbsp. butter, softened
- 1/2 tsp. black pepper
- 1/2 tsp. garlic powder
- 1/4 tsp. thyme, dried
- 1/4 tsp. oregano, dried

Directions:

1. Mix the turkey brine ingredients in a pot and soak the turkey in the brine overnight.
2. Next day, remove the soaked turkey from the brine.
3. Whisk the butter, black pepper, garlic powder, oregano, and thyme.
4. Brush the butter mixture over the turkey then place it in a baking tray.
5. Press "Power Button" of Air Fry Oven and turn the dial to select the "Air Roast" mode.
6. Now push the Temp button and rotate the dial to set the temperature at 370°F.
7. Once preheated, place the turkey baking tray in the oven and close its lid.
8. Slice and serve warm.

Nutrition: calories 383, fat 14g, fiber 4g, carbs 3g, protein 8g

Dinner:
Broccoli Soup, Green Leaves, and Beans

Preparation time: 10 minutes
Cooking time: 30 minutes
Servings: 2
Ingredients:

- 1 tbsp. of olive oil
- 1/2 medium size onion, cut into large pieces
- 3 cloves garlic in pieces
- 1 tsp. salt
- 1 medium size broccoli head in pieces
- 6 cups water
- 1 spinach bunches or 3 large fleas green leaves kale, spinach, etc.
- 1 fist cilantro leaves and stems
- 1 cup, Beans
- Dill (Optional)
- Lemon juice to serve

Directions:

1. Place a large pot and a lid over medium heat and add the tablespoon of olive oil, onion, garlic and half a teaspoon of salt. Leave for 5-7 minutes or until the onion is transparent.
2. Add water and spinach. Cover and let it begin to boil over low heat.
3. When the broccoli is soft add the cilantro fist, the dill (if you are going to use it) and the beans.
4. Blend very carefully with a food processor or in the blender. Check salt and add black pepper.
5. Before you serve, squeeze the juice of a lemon

Nutrition: calories 33, fat 1g, fiber 1g, carbs 6g, protein 2g

Day 3

Breakfast:

Green Beans Lunch Stew

Preparation time: 5 minutes
Cooking time: 15 minutes
Serving: 2
Ingredients:
- 1 pound green beans, halved
- 4 carrots, sliced
- 1 yellow onion, chopped
- 1 tbsp. thyme, chopped
- 3 tbsp. tomato paste
- Salt and black pepper to taste
- 4 garlic cloves, minced

Directions:
1. In a pan that fits your air fryer, place all the ingredients and toss until combined.
2. Place the pan in the air fryer and cook at 365°F for 15 minutes.
3. Divide the stew into bowls and serve.

Nutrition: calories 200, fat 8g, fiber 2g, carbs 8g, protein 6g

Snack
Kale Chips
Preparation time: 15 minutes
Cooking time: 55 minutes
Servings: 2
Ingredients:
- ¾ lb. kale
- ½ tsp. salt
- 1/8 tsp. sucralose sweetener
- 1 cup oil

Directions:
1. Set the Instant Pot to sauté.
2. Add the oil.
3. Once hot, fry the kale leaves.
4. Season with the salt and sweetener before serving.

Nutrition: calories 260, fat 25g, fiber 2g, carbs 8g, protein 2g

Lunch:

Easy Italian Meatballs

Preparation time: 10 minutes

Cooking Time: 13 minutes

Serving: 2

Ingredients:

- 2 lb. lean ground turkey
- ¼ cup onion, minced
- 2 cloves garlic, minced
- 2 tbsp. parsley, chopped
- 2 eggs
- 1½ cup parmesan cheese, grated

Directions:

1. Toss all the meatball ingredients in a bowl and mix well.
2. Make small meatballs out this mixture and place them in the air fryer basket.
3. Press "Power Button" of Air Fry Oven and turn the dial to select the "Air Fry" mode.
4. Press the Time button and again turn the dial to set the cooking time to 13 minutes.
5. Now push the Temp button and rotate the dial to set the temperature at 350°F.
6. Once preheated, place the air fryer basket inside and close its lid.
7. Flip the meatballs when cooked halfway through.
8. Serve warm.

Nutrition: calories 200, fat 8g, fiber 2g, carbs 8g, protein 6g

Dinner:
Celestial Seafood Gumbo

Preparation time: 10 minutes
Cooking time: 20 minutes
Servings: 2
Ingredients:

- 24 oz. sea bass fillets, cut into 2-inch pieces
- 2 pounds shrimp, peeled and deveined
- 4 tbsp. avocado oil
- 3 tbsp. Cajun seasoning
- 1 chopped ,Onion
- 1 Pepper
- 2 Celery
- 3 chopped ,Tomatoes
- 5 tbsp,Tomato Paste
- 3 bay leaves
- 1 ½ cup chicken broth
- 1 tsp. salt
- 1 tsp. black pepper

Directions:

1. Press the Sauté button and add the avocado oil to the Instant Pot.
2. Once the oil is hot, add the fish pieces and sauté until cooked through. Remove and set aside.
3. Add the onions, pepper, and celery and cook for 2 minutes or until softened, stirring occasionally.
4. Add the tomatoes, tomato paste, bay leaves and chicken broth.
5. Lock the lid and cook at high pressure for 5 minutes.
6. Press the Sauté button and stir in the shrimp, Cajun seasoning, salt, and black pepper. Cook just until the shrimp are cooked through, 3-5 mins.
7. Serve and enjoy!

Nutrition: calories 260, fat 8g, fiber 2g, carbs 8g, protein 45g

Day 4

Breakfast:

Healthy Green Beans

Preparation Time: 5 minutes
Cooking Time: 6 Minutes
Serving: 2
Ingredients:
- 1 lb green beans, trimmed
- 1tsb,Pepper
- 1 tbsp,Salt
- Cooking spray

Directions:
1. Spray air fryer basket with cooking spray.
2. Preheat the air fryer to 400°F.
3. Add green beans in air fryer basket and season with pepper and salt.
4. Cook green beans for 6 minutes. Turn halfway through.
5. Serve and enjoy.

Nutrition: calories 40, fat 1g, fiber 2g, carbs 8g, protein 2g

Snack
Cucumber with Tuna Flakes
Preparation time: 15 minutes
Cooking time: 20 minutes
Servings: 2
Ingredients:
- 12 round slices cucumber
- ½ cup canned tuna
- ¼ cup mayonnaise
- ½ onion, chopped
- 1 tsp. basil, dried

Directions:
1. Mix all the ingredients except the cucumber.
2. Top each cucumber round with the mixture.
3. Chill for a few minutes before serving.

Nutrition: calories 100, fat 7g, fiber 2g, carbs 8g, protein 6g

Lunch:
Butternut squash sauce
Preparation time: 10 minutes
cooking time: 13 minutes
servings: 12
Ingredients:
- 2 cups water
- ½ cup cashew, chopped
- 2 tbsp. olive oil
- 2 sweet onions, diced
- 2 tbsp. garlic, minced
- ½ tsp. salt
- ¼ cup dry white wine
- ¾ tsp. oregano, dried
- 1 cup butternut squash puree
- ⅛ tsp. ground nutmeg

Directions:
1. Blend cashews and water in a food processor until smooth. Set aside.
2. Pour the oil into a pan over medium heat.
3. Cook the onion and garlic for 3 minutes.
4. Season with salt.
5. Reduce heat and cook for another 10 minutes.
6. Stir in the wine and oregano.
7. Add the squash puree, nutmeg and cashew.
8. Cook for 3 minutes.
9. Refrigerate for up to 3 days

Nutrition: calories 200, fat 8g, fiber 2g, carbs 8g, protein 6g

Dinner:

Vegetarian Cauliflower Crust Pizza with Mushrooms and Olives

Preparation time: 10 minutes

Cooking time: 45 minutes

Servings: 2

Ingredients:

- 1 cup cauliflower, very finely chopped
- ½ cup low-fat mozzarella cheese, finely grated
- A pinch salt
- 1 egg, beaten

For your pizza topping:

- ¼ cup of tomato sauce
- 3 Mushrooms
- Almond meal
- ½ cup ,Parmesan cheese
- 1tbsp Oregano flakes
- 2tsp ,Garlic powder

Directions:

1. Heat the stove to 450°F/230°C.and sprinkle olive oil.
2. Now using a food processor, blender, or box grater, chop the cauliflower into bits that resemble rice.
3. Put the cauliflower in a safe microwave bowl and cook the cauliflower until it's completely softened (about 8 minutes). Do not add any water or liquid.
4. While you wait for the cauliflower to cook, slice your mushrooms and sauté them in a skillet with the olive oil. They should be well cooked and soft.
5. In a bowl, mix the cooked cauliflower were with the almond meal, Parmesan cheese, ½ cup of the finely grated mozzarella, oregano flakes, mushroom garlic powder and the pinch of salt. Beater the egg and add it to the other ingredients making sure to blend well.
6. Now spray a cookie sheet with nonstick cooking spray.
7. When your crust is ready, spread on the tomato sauce, sprinkle on the cheese, and distribute your sautéed mushrooms and olives evenly.

Nutrition: calories 200, fat 8g, fiber 2g, carbs 8g, protein 6g

Day 5

Breakfast:
Spicy & Tender Pork Chops

Preparation Time: 5 minutes
Cooking Time: 10 Minutes
Serving: 2
Ingredients:
- 4 pork chops
- 2 tsp. olive oil
- 1/2 tsp. dried sage
- 1 tbsp. Paprika
- 1 clove ,Garlic
- 1 tsp. Salt
- 1/2 tsp. cayenne pepper
- 1/4 tsp. pepper
- 1 tsp. ground cumin

Directions:
1. Preheat the air fryer to 400°F.
2. In a small bowl, mix together paprika, garlic salt, sage, pepper, cayenne pepper, and cumin.
3. Rub pork chops with spice mixture and place into the air fryer and cook for 10 minutes. Turn halfway through.
4. Serve and enjoy.

Nutrition: calories 275, fat 20g, fiber 2g, carbs 8g, protein 20g

Snack

Zucchini Crisps

Preparation time: 15 minutes
Cooking time: 35 minutes
Servings: 2
Ingredients:

- 2 medium zucchinis, sliced into rounds
- 2 tbsp. extra virgin olive oil
- Salt and pepper to taste
- 2 tbsp. Parmesan cheese, grated

Directions:

1. Add the oil to the Instant Pot.
2. Set it to sauté.
3. Fry the zucchini until golden.
4. Season with the salt, pepper and Parmesan.

Nutrition: calories 200, fat 8g, fiber 2g, carbs 8g, protein 6g

Lunch:
Comfort Soup
Preparation Time: 5 minutes
Cooking Time: 35 minutes
Serving: 3
Ingredients:
- ½ cups onion freshly diced
- 1 once Celery
- 2 carrots Carrot
- 1 tablespoon minced Garlic
- 1 tablespoon Curry powder
- 1 tsp. paprika
- ½ tbsp. water
- 3 ½ cups water
- ½ tsp. sea salt
- 1 tablespoon Freshly ground black pepper to taste
- ¼ tsp. dried thyme
- 1 lb,Lentils - A handful ,Rosemary
- 1 tsp. ,Vinegar

Directions:
1. Put a large pot on the stove over medium heat.
2. Add 1 ½ teaspoons of water along with celery, onion, carrot, paprika, garlic, curry powder, sea salt, black pepper, and thyme.
3. After all the herbs and spices are inside the pot, cover them and cook for about 7-8 minutes, stirring occasionally so that the spices do not burn.
4. Rinse the lentils and add them to 3 ½ cups of water. Stir into the stock.
5. Cover the pot and allow everything to simmer for 12-15 minutes.
6. Add the rosemary and simmer for another 10 minutes. You will know that your soup is ready when the lentils are fully softened.
7. Add the vinegar and some more water, if you want a thinner liquid.
8. Serve the soup with your favorite bread.

Nutrition: calories 200, fat 8g, fiber 2g, carbs 8g, protein 6g

Dinner:

Cream of Pear and Arugula

Preparation time: 10 minutes

Cooking time: 30 minutes

Servings: 2

Ingredients:

- ½ L Water
- 2 tsp., Extra virgin olive oil
- 4 pears blanquillos with leather, at its point of maturation
- 1 bowl arugula
- 2 tbsp. fresh aromatic herbs
- 1 small lemon, the juice
- 1 tsp., Sea salt or herbal salt
- 1 tsp. ,Pepper
- Edible flowers to decorate

Directions:

1. Grind all the ingredients inside the blender jar, except extra virgin olive oil and flowers, until a creamy and homogeneous texture is obtained. If necessary, rectify water, salt, and pepper.
2. Refrigerate until ready to serve and, once in the bowl, decorate with the flowers and a thread of olive oil. If you do not have flowers, you can use chopped almonds, some rocket leaves or sesame seeds.

To know more: The pear is a fruit with satiating effect for its fiber content: it is fantastic for people who want to lose weight and are doing a diet to lose weight.

Also, it is a fruit with anti-inflammatory action, helps us maintain a regular intestinal transit and combat constipation, and has a very beneficial effect on our microbiota or intestinal flora. Choose it whenever you can from organic farming.

Nutrition: calories 198, fat 12g, fiber 2g, carbs 20g, protein 5g

Day 6

Breakfast:
Spicy Catfish

Preparation Time: 15 minutes
Cooking Time: 13 minutes
Servings: 2

Ingredients:
- 2 tbsp. almond flour
- ½ tsp. paprika
- ½ tsp. garlic powder
- Salt, as required
- 2 (6-oz.) catfish fillets
- 1 tbsp. olive oil

Directions:
1. In a bowl, mix together the flour, paprika, garlic powder and salt.
2. Add the catfish fillets and coat with the mixture evenly.
3. Now, coat each fillet with oil.
4. Press "Power Button" of Air Fry Oven and turn the dial to select the "Air Fry" mode.
5. Press the Time button and again turn the dial to set the cooking time to 13 minutes.
6. Now push the Temp button and rotate the dial to set the temperature at 400°F.
7. Press "Start/Pause" button to start.
8. When the unit beeps to show that it is preheated, open the lid.
9. Arrange the fish fillets in greased "Air Fry Basket" and insert in the oven.
10. Flip the fish fillets once halfway through.

Nutrition: calories 340, fat 23g, fiber 2g, carbs 8g, protein 28g

Snack

Chicken Wings

Preparation time: 15 minutes
Cooking time: 25 minutes
Servings: 2
Ingredients:
- ½ serving all purpose low carb baking mix
- 2 tbsp. chili powder
- 1 tsp. cayenne pepper
- 2 tsp. yellow mustard seed
- 2 tsp. salt
- 12-16 chicken wings

Directions:
1. Preheat oven to 450°F
2. Rinse the chicken wings.
3. Line a baking sheet with aluminum foil. Spray with non-stick cooking spray.
4. Take a Ziploc bag, add the baking mix, chili powder, cayenne pepper, mustard seed, salt. Place the wings in the bag. Massage the chicken wings through the bag to coat them with seasoning.
5. Transfer to baking sheet. Cook 30-35 minutes, until golden brown.
6. Serve immediately.

Nutrition: calories 270, fat 18g, fiber 1g, carbs 3g, protein 22g

Lunch:
Lamb Tomato Bake
Preparation time: 10 minutes
Cooking Time: 35 minutes
Serving: 2
Ingredients:
- 25 oz. potatoes, boiled
- 14 oz. lean lamb mince
- 1 tsp. cinnamon
- 23 oz. jar tomato pasta

Sauce:
- 12 oz. white sauce
- 1 tbsp. olive oil

Directions:
1. Mash the potatoes in a bowl and stir in white sauce and cinnamon.
2. Sauté lamb mince with olive oil in a frying pan until brown.
3. Layer a casserole dish with tomato pasta sauce.
4. Top the sauce with lamb mince.
5. Spread the potato mash over the lamb in an even layer.
6. Press "Power Button" of Air Fry Oven and turn the dial to select the "Bake" mode.
7. Press the Time button and again turn the dial to set the cooking time to 35 minutes.
8. Now push the Temp button and rotate the dial to set the temperature at 350°F.
9. Once preheated, place casserole dish in the oven and close its lid.
10. Serve warm.

Nutrition: calories 350, fat 8g, fiber 2g, carbs 8g, protein 26g

Dinner:
Baked Brie with Tomatoes and Nuts

Preparation Time: 5 minutes

Cooking time: 10 minutes

Serving: 2

Ingredients:

- 8 oz. brie cheeses
- 1 tbsp. parsley, chopped
- 1 tbsp. sundried tomatoes, chopped
- ½ oz. pine nuts, dried

Directions:

1. Preheat the oven to 450°F.
2. Remove the white rind from the top of the cheese.
3. Put the cheese in a pie plate
4. Combine parsley and tomatoes together in a bowl. Mix well.
5. Distribute the tomato mixture evenly over the cheese. Sprinkle pine nuts on top.
6. Cook in the oven for about 10 minutes.

Nutrition: calories 200, fat 8g, fiber 2g, carbs 8g, protein 6g

Day 7
Breakfast:
Seasoned Catfish

Preparation Time: 15 minutes
Cooking Time: 23 minutes
Serving: 2
Ingredients:
- 4 (4-oz.) catfish fillets
- 2 tbsp. Italian seasoning
- Salt and ground black pepper, as required
- 1 tbsp. olive oil
- 1 tbsp. fresh parsley, chopped

Directions:
1. Rub the fish fillets with seasoning, salt and black pepper generously and then, coat with oil.
2. Press "Power Button" of Air Fry Oven and turn the dial to select the "Air Fry" mode.
3. Press the Time button and again turn the dial to set the cooking time to 20 minutes.
4. Now push the Temp button and rotate the dial to set the temperature at 400 degrees F.
5. Press "Start/Pause" button to start.
6. When the unit beeps to show that it is preheated, open the lid.
7. Arrange the fish fillets in greased "Air Fry Basket" and insert in the oven.
8. Flip the fish fillets once halfway through.
9. Serve hot with the garnishing of parsley.

Nutrition: calories 250, fat 8g, fiber 2g, carbs 8g, protein 17g

Snack
Smoked Chicken with Crepes Rolls
Preparation Time: 25 minutes
Cooking Time: 15 minutes
Servings: 2
Ingredients:
- 1 cup light cream cheese
- 4 slices (200g) smoked chicken
- 3 tsp. fresh dill, chopped
- 400g crepes, thawed
- 1½ tsp. lemon rind
- 1 small red onion, sliced
- 1 tsp. Salt and Pepper

Directions:
1. Add the cream cheese with lemon rind and dill in a mixing bowl.
2. Add salt and pepper and mix well.
3. Arrange the crepes onto a plate and add the cream cheese mixture on top generously.
4. Add 1 slice of the red onion followed by a slice of chicken.
5. Tightly roll them and seal the edges using a toothpick.
6. Repeat with the rest and serve fresh.

Nutrition: calories 185, fat 12g, fiber 2g, carbs 4g, protein 11g

Lunch:
French Quesadillas

Preparation Time: 10 minutes
Cooking time: 5 minutes
Serving: 2
Ingredients:
- 3 oz. boneless ham, cooked and sliced
- ¼ cup almonds, sliced
- 1 pear, sliced
- 4 oz. brie cheese, sliced
- 4 tortillas, low-carb

Directions:
1. Preheat your oven to 350°F
2. Arrange the tortillas on a sheet pan. Place pear slices on top of the tortillas followed by ham, cheese and almonds.
3. Fold the tortillas and cook for about 5 minutes.

Nutrition: calories 200, fat 8g, fiber 2g, carbs 8g, protein 6g

Dinner:
Carrot Nut Muffins
Preparation Time: 10 minutes
Cooking time: 25 minutes
Servings: 12
Ingredients:
- 1 cup whole grain soy flour
- 2 tsp. vanilla extract
- 1 ½ cups sweetener, sucralose-based
- 1 cup almond flour, blanched
- 2 tsp. cinnamon
- 1 cup carrots, grated
- ½ tsp. salt
- 1 cup vegetable oil
- 4 eggs
- ½ tsp. double acting baking powder, straight phosphate
- Non-stick cooking spray

Directions:
1. Preheat your oven to 350°F. Grease a 12-cup muffin tin using a non-stick cooking spray and set aside.
2. Combine soy flour, baking powder, almond flour, salt, sweetener and cinnamon together in a bowl.
3. Place remaining ingredients in a separate bowl and mix thoroughly.
4. Combine the two mixtures together until blended well. Pour equal amounts of the batter into the muffin tins. Cook in the oven for about 20-25 minutes.
5. Once done, place muffins in a wire rack to cool.

Nutrition: calories 280, fat 8g, fiber 2g, carbs 7g, protein 8g

ХНАПТЕР 5:

Meal Plan Day 8-14

Day 8

Breakfast:

Crispy Catfish

Preparation Time: 15 minutes
Cooking Time: 15 minutes
Servings: 5
Ingredients:

- 5 (6-oz.) catfish fillets
- 1 cup milk
- 2 tsp. fresh lemon juice
- ½ cup yellow mustard
- ½ cup cornmeal
- ¼ cup all-purpose flour
- 2 tbsp. dried parsley flakes
- ¼ tsp. red chili powder
- ¼ tsp. cayenne pepper
- ¼ tsp. onion powder
- ¼ tsp. garlic powder
- Salt and ground black pepper, as required
- Olive oil cooking spray

Directions:

1. In a large bowl, place the catfish, milk, and lemon juice and refrigerate for about 15 minutes.
2. In a shallow bowl, add the mustard.

3. In another bowl, mix together the cornmeal, flour, parsley flakes, and spices.
4. Remove the catfish fillets from milk mixture and with paper towels, pat them dry.
5. Coat each fish fillet with mustard and then, roll into cornmeal mixture.
6. Then, spray each fillet with the cooking spray.
7. Press "Power Button" of Air Fry Oven and turn the dial to select the "Air Fry" mode.
8. Now push the Temp button and rotate the dial to set the temperature at 400°F.
9. Press "Start/Pause" button to start.
10. When the unit beeps to show that it is preheated, open the lid.
11. Arrange the catfish fillets in greased "Air Fry Basket" and insert in the oven.
12. After 10 minutes of cooking, flip the fillets and spray with the cooking spray.

Nutrition: calories 340, fat 15g, fiber 2g, carbs 18g, protein 30g

Snack

Low-Carb Chicken Skewers

Preparation Time: 35 minutes
Cooking Time: 30 minutes
Servings: 4
Ingredients:

- 2 chicken breasts cut into medium chunks
- 2 carrots cut into thick circles
- 4 tbsp. soya sauce
- 1 tbsp. ginger garlic paste
- 1 tbsp. melted butter
- 4 tomatoes, thickly diced
- Salt and pepper to taste
- 8 onions, halved
- 1 tsp. lime juice

Directions:

1. In a bowl, combine the lime juice, pepper, soya sauce, butter, salt, and ginger garlic paste.
2. Add the chicken chunks and mix well.
3. Let it stand for about 30 minutes or longer.
4. Preheat your oven to 350°F and add aluminum foil to your baking sheet.
5. Now take your skewers and thread the chicken, tomato, onion, and carrot in a manner such that everything is in equal proportion.
6. Arrange them onto your baking sheet and bake in the oven for 15 minutes and serve with tomato sauce.

Nutrition: calories 200, fat 8g, fiber 2g, carbs 8g, protein 6g

Lunch:

Oregano Chicken Breast

Preparation time: 10 minutes
Cooking Time: 25 minutes
Serving: 2
Ingredients:

- 2 lbs. chicken breasts, minced
- 1 tbsp. avocado oil
- 1 tsp. smoked paprika
- 1 tsp. garlic powder
- 1 tsp. oregano
- 1/2 tsp. salt
- Black pepper, to taste

Directions:

1. Toss all the meatball ingredients in a bowl and mix well.
2. Make small meatballs out this mixture and place them in the air fryer basket.
3. Press "Power Button" of Air Fry Oven and turn the dial to select the "Air Fry" mode.
4. Press the Time button and again turn the dial to set the cooking time to 25 minutes.
5. Now push the Temp button and rotate the dial to set the temperature at 375°F.
6. Once preheated, place the air fryer basket inside and close its lid.

Nutrition: calories 354, fat 14g, fiber 2g, carbs 16g, protein 26g

Dinner:
Instant Pot Mussels and Crabs
Preparation Time: 10 Minutes
Cooking Time: 8 Minutes
Servings: 6
Ingredients:
- 6 tbsp. butter
- 2 shallots, chopped
- 1 tsp. of garlic, minced
- ½ cup white wine
- 2 lbs mussels, cleaned
- ½ lb of crab leg

Directions:
1. Wash and debeard mussels; throw away cracked mussels or mussels with shells that do not close.
2. Using the sauté mode, melt the butter in the Instant Pot.
3. Add the shallots; stirring frequently, cook until translucent.
4. Add the garlic and cook until aromatic. Approximately 1 minute.
5. Stir in the wine.
6. Add the mussels and crab.
7. Close the lid and lock it.
8. Set the vent to Sealing.
9. Cook on high pressure for 5 minutes.
10. When the timer beeps, naturally release the steam.
11. Open the lid.
12. Remove the mussels and crab to a serving platter.
13. Serve.

Nutrition: calories 3200, fat 8g, fiber 2g, carbs 0g, protein 34g

Day 9
Breakfast:
Air Fried Thyme Garlic Lamb Chops

Preparation Time: 5 minutes
Cooking Time: 12 Minutes
Serving: 2
Ingredients:
- 4 lamb chops
- 4 garlic cloves, minced
- 3 tbsp. olive oil
- 1 tbsp. dried thyme
- 1 tbsp. ,Pepper
- 1 tbsp. Salt

Directions:
1. Preheat the air fryer to 390°F.
2. Season lamb chops with pepper and salt.
3. In a small bowl, mix together thyme, oil, and garlic, and rub over lamb chops.
4. Place lamb chops into the air fryer and cook for 12 minutes. Turn halfway through.
5. Serve and enjoy

Nutrition: calories 415, fat 35g, fiber 2g, carbs 8g, protein 20g

Snack

Eggplant Stacks

Preparation Time: 20 minutes
Cooking Time: 5 minutes
Servings: 2
Ingredients:
- 4 oz. mozzarella cut into 8 slices
- 6½ tbsp. extra-virgin olive oil
- 1 tsp. oregano, dried
- ¼ cup pine nuts, toasted
- 1 tsp. salt
- 3 tbsp. balsamic vinegar
- 1 eggplant, cut into 1.2-cm circles
- 1 large garlic clove
- 1 cup basil leaves, packed
- 5/8 tsp. black pepper, ground
- ¼ cup parmesan cheese, grated
- 1 medium tomato, sliced

Directions:
1. In a large mixing bowl, combine the oil, salt, half of the vinegar, garlic, pepper, and oregano.
2. Mix well and add the eggplant slices.
3. Coat nicely and let it marinate for 10 minutes or longer.
4. In a griller, add the eggplants and grill for about 3 to 5 minutes.
5. Add the cheese, pine nuts, basil, and some water into a blender.
6. Blend until it is smooth.
7. Coat the tomato slices in salt, pepper, and vinegar.
8. Serve the eggplants with tomato slices and the cheese mixture.

Nutrition: calories 210, fat 8g, fiber 2g, carbs 8g, protein 7g

Lunch:

Roasted Squash

Preparation Time: 10 minutes
Cooking Time: 35 Minutes
Serving: 2
Ingredients:
- 4 cups butternut squash, diced
- 1/4 cup cranberries, dried
- 3 garlic cloves, minced
- 1 tbsp. soy sauce
- 1 tbsp. balsamic vinegar
- 1 tbsp. olive oil
- 8 oz. mushrooms, quartered
- 1 cup green onions, sliced

Directions:
1. In a large mixing bowl, mix together squash, mushrooms, and green onion and set aside.
2. In a small bowl, whisk together oil, garlic, vinegar, and soy sauce.
3. Pour oil mixture over squash and toss to coat.
4. Spray air fryer basket with cooking spray.
5. Add squash mixture into the air fryer basket and cook for 30-35 minutes at 400°F. Shake after every 5 minutes.
6. Toss with cranberries and serve hot.

Nutrition: calories 82, fat 4g, fiber 2g, carbs 14g, protein 3g

Dinner:
Burgundy Chicken

Preparation: 30 minutes
Cooking time: 60 minutes
Serving: 6
Ingredients:
- 4 tbsp. extra virgin olive oil
- 2 small onion, chopped
- 1 stalk celery, chopped
- 1 medium carrot, chopped
- 2 tsp. garlic
- 4 oz. boneless ham, cooked
- 2 lbs. chicken thigh
- 1 cup red table wine
- 1/2 cup chicken broth, organic and homemade
- 1 bay leaf - 2 tbsp. parsley, for garnishing

Directions:
1. Dice onion and ham; chop celery and carrot, and mince garlic.
2. Using large, heavy skillet heat 1 tablespoon oil.
3. Add onion, celery, and carrot; cook until the vegetables soften (approximately 5 minutes.)
4. Stir in garlic and ham; cook an additional 2 minutes.
5. Transfer to a bowl.
6. Heat the rest of the oil; brown the chicken on all sides.
7. Stir in the wine, broth, and bay leaf.
8. Reduce heat: cook until the chicken is completely cooked and most of the liquid reduced Stir the ham and vegetables into the chicken mixture; heat for approximately 5 minutes.
9. Remove the bay leaf; place chicken in a serving bowl.
10. Sprinkle with parsley, if desired.
11. Serve.

Nutrition: calories 450, fat 8g, fiber 22g, carbs 8g, protein 43g

Day 10

Breakfast:

Greek Chicken

Preparation Time: 10 minutes
Cooking Time: 24 Minutes
Serving: 2
Ingredients:
- 2 lbs. chicken tenders
- 1 cup cherry tomatoes
- 2 tbsp. olive oil
- 3 dill sprigs
- 1 large zucchini

For topping:
- 2 tbsp. feta cheese, crumbled
- 1 tbsp. fresh dill, chopped
- 1 tbsp. olive oil
- 1 tbsp. fresh lemon juice

Directions:
1. Preheat the air fryer to 370°F.
2. Spray air fryer basket with cooking spray.
3. Add chicken, zucchini, dill, and tomatoes into the air fryer basket. Drizzle with olive oil and season with salt.
4. Cook chicken for 24 minutes.
5. Meanwhile, in a small bowl, stir together all topping ingredients.
6. Place chicken on the serving plate then top with veggies and discard dill sprigs.
7. Sprinkle topping mixture on top of chicken and vegetables.
8. Serve and enjoy.

Nutrition: calories 555, fat 28g, fiber 2g, carbs 6g, protein 67g

Snack
Zucchini Fritters

Preparation Time: 10 minutes
Cooking Time: 5 minute
Servings: 4
Ingredients:

- 3 medium zucchinis, peeled and grated
- ½ cup parmesan, finely grated
- 1 tsp. salt
- 3 shallots, thinly sliced
- ¼ cup fresh parsley, chopped
- ½ cup low-carb flour
- 1 egg, whisked
- 2 tsp. dried oregano leaves
- 4 tsp. olive oil
- ¼ tsp. ground nutmeg

Directions:

1. In a large mixing bowl, combine the grated zucchini with shallots.
2. Add the low-carb flour, cheese, nutmeg, salt, and oregano.
3. Beat in an egg and mix well.
4. Create flat fritters using your hands.
5. In a skillet, add the olive oil and heat over medium heat.
6. Fry the fritters golden brown from both sides.
7. Serve with any sauce or with lettuce leaves.

Nutrition: calories 200, fat 8g, fiber 2g, carbs 8g, protein 6g

Lunch:

Beef Roast

Preparation Time: 10 minutes
Cooking Time: 45 Minutes
Serving: 2
Ingredients:

- 2 1/2 lbs beef roast
- 1 tsp. onion powder
- 1 tsp. rosemary
- 1 tsp. dill
- 2 tbsp. olive oil
- 1/4 tsp. pepper
- 1 tsp. garlic powder

Directions:

1. Preheat the air fryer to 360°F.
2. Mix together pepper, garlic powder, onion powder, rosemary, dill, and oil. Rub all over the beef roast.
3. Place roast in the air fryer and cook for 45 minutes.
4. Serve and enjoy.

Nutrition: calories 294, fat 12g, fiber 2g, carbs 8g, protein 45g

Dinner:
Minced Chicken
Preparation Time: 10 minutes
Cooking Time: 35 Minutes
Serving: 2
Ingredients:
- 2 tbsp. olive oil
- 1 tsp. cumin seeds
- 1/6 tsp. turmeric
- 1 tbsp. garlic, grated
- 2 tbsp. ginger, grated
- 1 large yellow onion, diced
- 4 tomatoes, diced
- 2 tsp. mild red chili powder
- 1 tsp. Garam Masala
- ¼ tsp. salt
- 1 tbsp. coriander powder
- 2 lbs ground chicken meat, boneless and skinless
- ½ cup water
- ½ cup cilantro, chopped for garnish

Directions:
1. Heat the oil using the sauté mode of the Instant Pot.
2. Add the cumin seeds and cook for 50 seconds.
3. Stir in the turmeric.
4. Add the ginger and garlic; stir until combined.
5. Stir in the onion; cook for 1 minute.
6. Cover with glass lid; cook for 2 minutes.
7. Open the pot; add the tomatoes, red chili powder, Garam Masala, salt, and coriander; stir until combined. Add the chicken; break it up using a spatula.
8. Stir in ½ cup of water. Close the lid and lock it.
9. Garnish with cilantro and serve.

Nutrition: calories 540, fat 8g, fiber 2g, carbs 8g, protein 67g

Day 11

Breakfast:
Salad with Avocado, Pineapple and Cucumbers

Preparation Time: 10 minutes
Cooking Time: 24 Minutes
Serving: 2
Ingredients:
- 1 cucumber, sliced
- 3 slices pineapple
- 1/2 red onion, filleted
- 2 avocados
- 1/3 cup olive oil
- 2 tbsp. lemon juice
- 1 tsp. salt
- 1 tsp. pepper

Direction:
1. Cut the avocado and pineapple in medium cubes.
2. Subsequently cut the cucumber along, remove the seeds with a spoon and cut into slices.
3. Mix the above in a bowl, add the red onion, salt, pepper and season with olive oil and lemon
4. Serve

Nutrition: calories 90, fat 4g, fiber 2g, carbs 8g, protein 6g

Snack

Coconut Orange Creamsicle Fat Bombs

Preparation time: 10 minutes
Cooking time: 20 minutes
Servings: 2
Ingredients:

- ½ cup coconut oil
- ½ cup heavy whipping cream
- ¼ cup cream cheese
- 1 tsp. orange vanilla Mio
- 10 drops liquid Stevia

Direction:

1. Add the coconut oil to a blender. Pulse until smooth.
2. Add the whip cream. Pulse until combined.
3. Add the cream cheese. Pulse until smooth.
4. Add the orange Milo and Stevia. Pulse until smooth.
5. Spoon the mixture into silicon tray mold or ice cube tray. Freeze 3 hours.
6. Pop out to eat. Store uneaten bombs in a bag in the freezer.
7. Serve

Nutrition: calories 200, fat 8g, fiber 2g, carbs 8g, protein 6g

Lunch:

Roasted Eggplant

Preparation Time: 10 minutes
Cooking Time: 12 Minutes
Servings: 2
Ingredients:

- 1 eggplant, washed and cubed
- 1/2 tsp. garlic powder
- 1/4 tsp. marjoram
- 1/4 tsp. oregano
- 1 tbsp. olive oil

Directions:

1. Spray air fryer basket with cooking spray.
2. Add all ingredients into the mixing bowl and toss well.
3. Transfer eggplant mixture into the air fryer basket and cook at 390°F for 6 minutes.
4. Toss well and cook for 6 minutes more.
5. Serve and enjoy.

Nutrition: calories 120, fat 8g, fiber 2g, carbs 12g, protein 3g

Dinner:
Turkey with Seasoning and Gravy

Preparation Time: 25 Minutes
Cooking Time: 45 Minutes
Servings: 2
Ingredients:
- 2 turkey breasts, boneless, skin on, tied with butcher twine
- 3 tbsp. butter, softened
- 1/3 cup lime Juice
- ½ cup of water

Seasoning Ingredients:
- 1/2 tsp. fresh thyme
- 2 tsp. fresh sage, chopped
- 1 1/3 tsp. salt - 1/4 tsp. smoked paprika
- 1/4 tsp. garlic salt

For The Gravy:
- ½ cup Drippings from the turkey
- 2 tbsp. tapioca starch - 3 tbsp. Water

Directions:
1. Whisk together the butter and seasoning Ingredients in a small bowl.
2. Spread ½ of the butter mixture under the skin and on the bottom of the turkey breast; the other half is spread on top of the skin.
3. Turn on the Instant Pot to sauté mode. Place the turkey, skin side down, in the Instant Pot.
4. Cook the turkey until golden brown; remove from the pot.
5. Place a trivet in the pot; add the water and lime juice.
6. Put the turkey on the trivet. Close the lid and lock it.
7. Set the vent to Sealing. Cook on high pressure for 35 minutes.
8. When the timer beeps, naturally release the steam for 10-15 minutes.
9. Serve the gravy with the turkey.

Nutrition: calories 200, fat 8g, fiber 2g, carbs 8g, protein 6g

Day 12

Breakfast:

Tuna Tartare with Avocado and Sesame

Preparation Time: 10 minutes
Cooking Time: 24 Minutes
Serving: 2
Ingredients:

- 300 gr fresh tuna
- 1/2 red onion - chopped
- 1 avocado
- 2 tsp. Juice of a lemon slice
- 1 tsp. sesame oil
- 1/2 Salt and Pepper
- 1 tbsp. roasted sesame seeds + extra for it
- Few sprigs fresh dill
- 2 tsps. sour cream
- Optional: four toasted slices of baguette for it

Directions:

1. Cut the tuna into very small cubes. Do the same with the avocado.
2. Take a large bowl and then mix the tuna, avocado, lemon juice, sesame seeds, red onion and sesame oil — season with a pinch of pepper and salt.
3. Place the ring on a plate and add half of the tuna mixture. Press with a spoon and carefully slide the ring off. Make the second steak tart as well.
4. Sprinkle some sesame seeds over the tartare and close with a teaspoon of sour cream and dill on each tuna tartare.

Nutrition: calories 210g, fat 12g, fiber 2g, carbs 8g, protein 6g

Snack

Protein Pancakes

Preparation Time: 5 minutes

Cooking time: 10

Servings: 4

Ingredients:

- 1 tbsp. vanilla whey protein
- ¼ cup almond meal
- 3 tbsp. whole grain soy flour
- 1 tsp. baking powder
- 3 large sized whole eggs
- ⅓ cup cottage cheese, creamed
- Butter for Cook

Direction:

1. In a bowl, combine almond meal, protein powder, baking powder and soy flour. Stir.
2. In a separate bowl, whisk the eggs. Add the creamed cottage cheese. Stir until combined. Add to dry ingredients. Stir until combined.
3. On a large griddle/skillet, melt butter over surface. Scoop out ¼ cup of batter. Cook 2-3 minutes per side, until golden brown.

Nutrition: calories 191, fat 9g, fiber 2g, carbs 8g, protein 20g

Lunch:
Curried Eggplant Slices

Preparation Time: 10 minutes
Cooking Time: 10 Minutes
Servings: 2
Ingredients:
- 1 large eggplant, cut into 1/2-inch thick slices
- 1 garlic clove, minced
- 1 tbsp. olive oil
- 1/2 tsp. curry powder
- 1/8 tsp. turmeric
- 1/2 tsp. Salt

Directions:
1. Preheat the air fryer to 300°F.
2. Add all ingredients into the large mixing bowl and toss to coat.
3. Transfer eggplant slices into the air fryer basket.
4. Cook eggplant slices for 10 minutes or until lightly brown. Shake basket halfway through.
5. Serve and enjoy.

Nutrition: calories 170, fat 8g, fiber 2g, carbs 8g, protein 4g

Dinner:

Low Carb Buffalo Chicken Wings

Preparation time: 10 minutes
Cooking time: 30 minutes
Servings: 6
Ingredients:

- 2 large eggs, (whole)
- 1 cup apple cider vinegar
- Salt, to taste
- 1/3 cup olive oil
- Black pepper, to taste
- 1 tsp. garlic powder - 1 tsp. celery salt
- ¼ tsp. cayenne pepper
- 3 lbs. chicken wing with, bone and skin

Dipping Ingredients:

- 16 tbsp. mayonnaise - ½ cup sour cream, cultured
- 3 medium scallions - ½ cup blue cheese, crumbled
- 1 fluid oz. lemon juice - 2 garlic cloves, minced

Directions:
Wings:

1. Preheat oven to 440°F.
2. In a medium bowl beat the egg; then, whisk together the egg, vinegar, olive oil, salt, pepper, garlic powder, celery salt, and cayenne.
3. Dip chicken wings into the marinade until thoroughly coated; arrange on a large baking sheet. Bake for approximately 30 minutes (until the wings are crisp); turn over and brush with marinade several times.

Dipping Sauce:

1. Dice scallions and minced garlic.
2. Mix mayonnaise, sour cream, blue cheese, scallions, lemon juice, and garlic; set aside.
3. Serve wings immediately after removing from the oven with the dipping sauce

Nutrition: calories 800, fat 8g, fiber 2g, carbs 12g, protein 69g

Day 13

Breakfast:
Low-Carb Chicken Breasts with Creamy Sauce

Preparation Time: 15 minutes
Cooking Time: 15 minutes
Serving: 2
Ingredients:

- 1 tsp. Lemon pepper
- 1/2 Salt
- 1 tsp. Dried dill weed
- 3 tsp. Butter
- ½ cup whipping cream
- 1 tsp. Garlic powder
- 4 chicken breasts
- 2 tbsp. capers, rinsed

Directions:

1. Get rid of the bones of the chicken breasts carefully.
2. Discard the skin and cut each chicken breast in half.
3. In a zipper bag, add the garlic powder, dried dill weed, salt, and pepper and add a little water to make a good marinating mixture.
4. Add the chicken breasts into the zipper bag.
5. Lock the zipper bag and shake it to coat the chicken breasts in the spice mixture.
6. Put it in the refrigerator for 30 to 50 minutes or longer.
7. Take a skillet and melt the butter over medium heat.
8. Add the chicken breasts and cook on both sides until they get a nice golden texture. Keep tossing the chicken breasts to make sure they are cooked through evenly. Once done, take off the heat.
9. To make the creamy sauce, add the whipping cream to a pan.
10. Stir for about 4 minutes; make sure it does not get burned.
11. Turn off the heat and add the capers. Mix well.

12. Serve the hot chicken breasts with a generous amount of creamy sauce on top.

Nutrition: calories 150, fat 7g, fiber 2g, carbs 8g, protein 10g

Snack
Corndog Muffins

Preparation time: 10 minutes
Cooking time: 15 minutes
Servings: 2
Ingredients:

- ½ cup blanched almond flour
- ½ cup flaxseed meal
- 1 tbsp. psyllium husk powder
- 3 tbsp. swerve sweetener
- ¼ tsp. salt
- ¼ tsp. baking powder
- ¼ cup butter, melted
- 1 egg
- ¼ cup coconut milk
- ⅓ cup sour cream
- 3 all beef hot dogs

Directions:

1. Preheat oven to 375°F
2. In a bowl, add the almond flour, flaxseed, husk powder, granulated sweetener, salt, and baking powder. Whisk together.
3. In a separate bowl, combine the egg, coconut milk. Whisk together. Add the butter. Stir until combined. Add the sour cream. Stir until combined.
4. Add the dry ingredients to the wet ingredients. Stir until a smooth batter forms.
5. Grease a 12 mini muffin tin.
6. Slice the hot dogs into 4 sections.
7. Fill the muffin cup half way. Add the sliced hot dog to the batter.
8. Bake 12 minutes.
9. Then broil 1-2 minutes, until golden brown. Serve.

Nutrition: calories 78, fat 8g, fiber 2g, carbs 8g, protein 6g

Lunch:
Yummy Cheesy Roasted Brussels
Preparation time: 5 Minutes
Cooking time: 20 Minutes
Serving: 2
Ingredients:
- ½ lb. Brussels sprouts, chopped
- ½ tbsp. olive oil
- 1 clove garlic, peeled and crushed
- ¼ tsp. fresh thyme, chopped
- 2 oz. cream cheese
- 1/8 cup sour cream
- 1/8 cup mayonnaise
- ½ cup mozzarella cheese, shredded
- 1/8 cup parmesan cheese, grated
- Salt and pepper to taste

Directions:
1. Literally toss all the ingredients into the cooker (trust us!).
2. Cover the cooker and cook for 1-2 hours on Low. It's done when the cheese is nice and melted.

Nutrition: calories 33, fat 8g, fiber 2g, carbs 8g, protein 13g

Dinner:
Cherry Tomato Chicken Cacciatore

Preparation time: 15 Minutes
Cooking time: 25 Minutes
Servings: 2
Ingredients:
- 1 lb. (500g) cherry tomatoes
- 1 tsp. salt
- 1 cup water
- 1 sprig fresh basil leaves, torn
- 2 garlic cloves, crushed.
- ¼ tsp. hot pepper flakes
- 1 tsp. olive oil
- 3 lb. bone-in chicken legs and thighs
- 1 tsp. dried oregano
- ¼ cup tart red table wine
- ½ cup (70g) pitted green olives, rinsed

Directions:
1. In the heated pressure cooker, heat the olive oil and brown the chicken thighs on all sides. In the meantime, remove the stems from the cherry tomatoes and place them in a big zip lock pack, so they are in a single layer.
2. Close the pack totally - leave a tiny opening at the end. Alternatively, on the other lightly tie a standard plastic bag. With a meat pounder or heavy pot, softly squash all part of the cherry tomatoes - the aim is to burst them open, not crush them.
3. Put the chicken aside and pour the pounded cherry tomato blend and the more significant part of its sap into the pressure cooker base.
4. Include the garlic, hot pepper, salt, oregano, wine, and water and blend well, scraping up the brown bits of chicken adhered to the bottom of the cooker.
5. Place the chicken over into the pressure cooker and blend to coat the chicken with the contents of the cooker. At that point, "smooth" out the chicken pieces into an even layer.

For stovetop pressure cookers:

1. Turn the heat up to high, and when the cooker indicates it has achieved high pressure, lower to the heat to continue it and begin counting 12 minutes pressure cooking time.

2. At the point when time is up, open the cooker by freeing the pressure through the valve.

3. Mix the contents and let the cooker stand unlidded for about 5 minutes, infrequently stirring to lessen some of the cooking fluid using the pressure cooker's lingering heat.

4. Using a slotted spoon, lift into a serving casserole and sprinkle with green olives and basil before serving. Keep the broth left in the base of the pressure cooker to use set up of stock in a risotto or rice recipe.

Nutrition: calories 280, fat 8g, fiber 3g, carbs 8g, protein 6g

Day 14

Breakfast:

Delicious Low-Carb Butter Chicken

Preparation Time: 15 minutes
Cooking Time: 45 minutes
Serving: 2
Ingredients:

- ½ tsp. Garlic
- 1 tsp. Salt
- 4 chicken breasts
- 1 tsp. paprika
- 1 tsp. oregano
- 1 cup crushed cracker crumbs
- 1/2 black pepper
- 2 eggs, - ½ cup butter stick

Directions:

1. Use a sharp knife to discard the skin of the chicken breasts.
2. Cut the chicken breasts in halves and set aside.
3. Cut the butter stick into smaller pieces and set aside.
4. Preheat the oven to 375°F.
5. Add parchment paper to your baking tray and set it aside.
6. In a mixing bowl, whisk the eggs until they become fluffy.
7. Take a plate and arrange the crushed cracker crumbs.
8. Sprinkle the garlic salt and ground black pepper onto the cracker crumbs.
9. Mix well and set aside. Now season the chicken with paprika and oregano. You can add a little salt, too.
10. Let the chicken sit for 10 minutes. Dip each chicken piece in the beaten egg mixture. Roll them on the cracker crumb mixture.
11. Bake in the preheated oven for about 45 minutes.
12. Let it cool down for 10 minutes before removing from the oven.
13. Serve with fresh lemon wedges. You can add any creamy sauce on the side.

Nutrition: calories 170, Fat 5g, Protein 8g, Carbs 7g

Snack
Almond and Coconut Mug Muffin

Preparation Time: 3 minutes

cooking time: 30 minutes

Servings: 6

Ingredients:
- 2 tbsp. almond flour
- ⅓ tbsp. Sucralose-based sweetener
- ⅓ tbsp. organic high fiber coconut flour
- ¼ tsp. almonds, minced
- Pinch dried coconut
- ½ tsp. Cinnamon
- ¼ tsp. baking powder
- ⅛ tsp. salt
- 1 large egg
- 1 tsp. extra virgin olive oil

Direction:
1. In a larger coffee mug, add the almond flour, sweetener, coconut flour, minced almond, dried coconut, cinnamon, baking powder, salt. Stir with a fork.
2. Crack in the egg. Pour in olive oil. Stir until combined.
3. Pop into the microwave. Cook for 1 minute. Cook at 15 second intervals if more time required.
4. Top with butter and more minced almond. Use a spoon to dig out the goodness

Nutrition: calories 207, fat 8g, fiber 2g, carbs 8g, protein 6g

Lunch:
Heavenly Braised Cabbage

Preparation time: 5 Minutes
Cooking time: 20 Minutes
Serving: 2
Ingredients:
- 1 head green cabbage
- 1 large sweet onion, sliced
- ¼-½ cup bone broth
- Sea salt to taste
- ¼ cup bacon fat, melted
- 4 garlic cloves, coarsely chopped (optional)

Directions:
1. Turn the cooker on High. Add onion and bacon into the cooker and cook, uncovered, until the fat has melted off the bacon.
2. Layer the cabbage pieces on top of the bacon-onion mixture.
3. Pour in the broth and add salt to taste.
4. Let the ingredients cook for an hour on High.
5. Stir the ingredients and continue cooking on High for no more than 4 hours.
6. Once done, drizzle some vinegar overtop and season with salt & pepper.
7. The cabbage is delicious served hot, and even better reheated the next day!

Nutrition: calories 108, fat 8g, fiber 2g, carbs 8g, protein 7g

Dinner:
Scrumptious Chicken Bacon Chowder

Preparation time: 5 Minutes
Cooking time: 20 Minutes
Serving: 2
Ingredients:

- 1 tsp. dried thyme
- 1 tsp. black pepper
- 1 tsp. sea salt
- 8 oz. cream cheese
- 1 medium sweet onion, thinly sliced
- 1 lb. chicken breasts or thighs
- 1 cup heavy cream
- 2 ribs celery, diced
- 1 tsp. garlic powder
- 2 cups chicken stock, divided
- 1 small leek, cleaned, trimmed and sliced
- 6 mushrooms, sliced
- 1 shallot, finely chopped
- 4 cloves garlic, minced
- 4 tbsp. butter, divided

Directions:

1. Turn the cooker on Low. Add the leeks, black pepper, mushrooms, onions, 1 cup chicken stock, sea salt, 2 tbsp. butter, shallot, celery and garlic into the cooker and stir to combine. Cover and cook for about 30 mins.
2. Heat 2 tbsp. butter in a frying pan over medium heat and pan-sear the chicken breasts until browned on both sides. Set aside.
3. Add the remaining 1 cup of chicken stock to the slow cooker. Add the thyme, heavy cream, cream cheese, and garlic powder into the slow cooker. Carefully stir the ingredients.

Nutrition: calories 340, fat 8g, fiber 2g, carbs 8g, protein 6g

ХНАПТЕР 6:

Meal Plan Day 15-21

Day 15

Breakfast:

Beef and Bacon Meatloaf with Brussels sprouts And Carrots

Preparation time: 10 Minutes

Cooking time: 35 Minutes

Serving: 2

Ingredients:

- 1 onion, finely chopped
- 2 tbsp. butter
- 25 oz. ground beef
- 1 egg
- ½ cup heavy whipping cream
- 1 tbsp. dried oregano
- 1 tsp. salt
- ½ cup cheese, shredded
- ½ tsp. pepper
- 7 oz. sliced bacon
- 1 ¼ cups heavy whipping cream for gravy

Directions:

1. Preheat the oven to 400°F.
2. In a pan, fry the chopped onion in butter until translucent and tender.
3. In a bowl, mix the ground beef, onions, egg, oregano, salt, heavy whipping cream, cheese, and pepper. Blend the ingredients gently together combining well.

4. Form the combination into a loaf shape and place in a baking dish or loaf pan.
5. Now wrap the loaf with the bacon slices.
6. Bake the bacon-wrapped loaf in the oven for forty-five to fifty minutes.
7. Should the bacon appear to overcook, you can cover the baking dish with some aluminum foil.
8. Pour the juices from the baking plate into a saucepan and add in 1 ¼ cups of heavy whipping cream.
9. Once the gravy boils, set the heat lower and simmer for 15 minutes.
10. Serve with gravy.

Nutrition: calories 108, fat 50g, fiber 2g, carbs 8g, protein 48g

Snack

Layered Fried Queso Blanco

Preparation time: 10 minutes
Cooking time: 20 minutes
Servings: 8
Ingredients:

- ½ cup Queso Blanco
- 1½ tbsp. olive oil
- Pinch red pepper flakes or salt and pepper

Directions:

1. Cut the cheese into cubes. Chill in the freezer as you heat the oil.
2. In a skillet, heat the olive oil. Once the pan is hot, add the cubes of cheese.
3. As it cooks it will melt. Once it is golden brown on one side, flip it over. Press down against the cheese to flatten it slightly and push out the oil. Once it is golden brown on both sides, tilt the edges against the pan and cook those until golden brown. It will seal the cheese into a square.
4. Remove from pan. Place on paper towel. Pat lightly. Slice into cubes again.
5. Sprinkle red pepper flakes or salt and pepper over the cubes. Serve immediately.

Nutrition: calories 200, fat 8g, fiber 2g, carbs 8g, protein 6g

Lunch:
Pressure Cooker Mussels in Spicy Tomato Sauce

Preparation Time: 15 Minutes

Cooking Time: 5-6minutes

Servings: 6

Ingredients:
- 4 tbsp. olive oil
- 2 large yellow onions, peeled and chopped
- 1 tsp. garlic, minced
- 1 tsp. red pepper flakes
- 16 oz. of tomatoes
- 1/3 cups chicken broth
- 2 tsp. dried oregano
- 2.5 lbs. mussels, scrubbed

Directions:
1. Using the sauté mode of instant pot, heat the oil.
2. Add the yellow onions and cook them until they are soft (approximately 3 minutes.)
3. Stir in the garlic and red pepper flakes; stir constantly for 20 seconds.
4. Add the tomatoes, chicken broth, and oregano; stir to combine.
5. Increase heat to a simmer.
6. Stir in the mussels; make sure they are completely covered in the sauce.
7. Close the lid and lock it.
8. Set the vent to Sealing.
9. Cook on high pressure for 1 minute.
10. When the timer beeps, quickly release the steam.
11. Open the lid.
12. Stir well and remove to a serving bowl.
13. Serve.

Nutrition: calories 150, fat 8g, fiber 2g, carbs 8g, protein 24g

Dinner:
Baked Pear Fans

Preparation Time: 10 minutes
Cooking time: 40
Servings: 4
Ingredients:
- 2 medium pears
- 1 tbsp. unsalted butter
- ¼ tsp. black pepper
- ¼ tsp. ginger
- ¼ tsp. cinnamon
- 1 tsp. tap water
- 2 tsp. Lemon Juice
- ¼ tsp. pure vanilla extract

Direction:
1. Preheat oven to 375°F
2. You are going to make fans out of your pears. Make ¼ inch slices along the length of your half pear, starting ⅓ of an inch from the stem while cutting them all the way down to the bottom.
3. In a skillet, melt the butter. Add the lemon juice and water. Stir in the ginger, pepper, and cinnamon.
4. Place the pears in the skillet.
5. Cover with aluminum foil. Transfer skillet to oven. Bake 40 minutes. Turn the pears halfway through cooking.
6. Using a slotted spoon, transfer pears to serving plates.
7. Place skillet on stove. Stir in the vanilla. Simmer 1 minute.
8. Scoop the sauce over the pears. Serve.

Nutrition: calories 200, fat 8g, fiber 2g, carbs 8g, protein 6g

Day 16

Breakfast:

Good Morning Atkins Waffles

Preparation Time: 10 minutes
Cooking Time: 20 minutes
Servings: 5
Ingredients:

- 1 large egg (whole)
- 1 pack sucralose based sugar substitute
- 2 tsp. baking powder
- 1 cup cream
- ½ tsp. salt
- 3 serving's soy flour, whole grain

Directions:

1. In a large bowl, add 1 cup soy flour, salt, sugar substitute, and baking powder. Blend the ingredients and mix well.
2. In another bowl, whisk the whole egg together with cream.
3. Add liquid ingredients to the dry ingredients and beat the batter well until there are no more lumps. Make sure you do not overbeat the mixture.
4. In order to activate the baking powder, allow the mixture to sit for at least 5 minutes.
5. In the meantime, heat the waffle iron and add the batter in the center of the iron.
6. Gently, close the top and let the waffles cook for 2 minutes or until they turn golden brown in color.

Nutrition: calories 163, fat 8g, fiber 2g, carbs 8g, protein 11g

Snack
Raspberry Lemon Popsicles
Preparation time: 10 minutes
Cooking time: 60 minutes
Servings: 6
Ingredients:
- 1 cup raspberries
- Juice from ½ a lemon
- ¼ cup coconut oil
- 1 cup coconut milk
- ¼ cup sour cream
- ¼ cup heavy cream
- ½ tsp. Guar Gum
- 20 drops liquid Stevia

Directions:
1. Combine all the ingredients in a blender. Pulse until smooth. Strain the liquid.
2. Pour mixture into popsicle molds. Freeze 2 hours.
3. If stuck, run the mold under hot water briefly

Nutrition: calories 200, fat 8g, fiber 2g, carbs 8g, protein 6g

Lunch:
Caramelized Pear Custard
Preparation time: 10 minutes
Cooking time: 20 minutes
Servings: 8
Ingredients:

- 2 tbsp. butter
- 2 tbsp. Xylitol
- ¼ tsp. cardamom, ground
- 2 medium pears
- 1/8 cup sugar-free low calorie maple syrup
- ½ tsp. rum

Directions:
1. Preheating oven to 375°F
2. Peel the pears. Slice them in half.
3. In a sauce pan, over medium heat, melt the butter. Add the rum, xylitol and cardamom. Stir well.
4. Add the pears to sauce pan. Cover with sauce. Cook 4 minutes per side.
5. Transfer the pears and sauce to a deep glass dish.
6. Bake 20 minutes, until golden brown and the custard has set.
7. Remove from oven. Cool slightly before serving.
8. Using a pastry brush, lightly brush the pears with maple syrup. Serve.

Nutrition: calories 200, fat 8g, fiber 1g, carbs 8g, protein 23g

Dinner:
Chocolate Brownie Drops

Preparation Time: 15 minutes
cooking time: 15 minutes
Servings: 12
Ingredients:

- ⅛ cup stone ground whole wheat pastry flour
- 2 tbsp. whole grain soy flour
- ¼ tsp. baking powder
- ¼ cup unsweetened chocolate baking squares
- 6 tbsp. heavy cream
- 2 tbsp. unsalted butter
- 2 large eggs
- ¾ cup sucralose based sweetener

Direction:

1. Preheat oven to 375°F
2. Microwave the chocolate squares until almost melted. Add the butter. Stir until shinny. Set aside to cool.
3. Line a baking sheet with parchment paper.
4. In a large bowl, using an electric mixer, blend the butter until smooth. Add the sugar substitute. Blend again until smooth. Add the eggs, one at a time. Continue beating until smooth. Add the cooled chocolate to bowl. Continue beating.
5. In a separate bowl, whisk the flour, baking powder, and soy flour.
6. Pour in the flour mixture slowly. Beat until just combined.
7. Using a rounded spoon, spoon drops of batter onto the baking sheet.
8. Bake 5-6 minutes. Transfer to wire rack to cool. Serve.

Nutrition: calories 104, fat 8g, fiber 2g, carbs 8g, protein 2.5g

Day 17

Breakfast:
Breakfast Tacos

Preparation time: 10 minutes
Cooking time: 40 minutes
Servings: 4
Ingredients:

- 1 cup mozzarella cheese, shredded
- 6 eggs
- 2 tbsp. butter
- 3 strips bacon
- ½ an avocado, thinly sliced
- ½ cup cheddar cheese, shredded
- Pinch salt and pepper

Directions:

1. Preheat oven to 375°F
2. Cook the bacon. Set aside.
3. You are going to make your very own cheese taco shells. Suspend a yard stick/ruler/long spoon between two items that prop it 6 inches from a counter.
4. Heat a skillet. Scoop half a cup of mozzarella cheese on the surface. Spread into a circle. Cook for 3 minutes until golden brown. Flip cook on other side. Lift the circle of cheese off surface, drape it over yardstick/ruler. Let it cool as you cook the others and rest of ingredients.
5. In a separate bowl, whisk the eggs. Season with salt and pepper. Melt butter in a skillet. Scramble the eggs.
6. Prepare the tacos: Place a slice of bacon in cheese taco shell. Add a couple spoons of cooked egg. Top with shredded cheddar cheese and sliced avocado.

Nutrition: calories 443, fat 8g, fiber1g, carbs 8g, protein 3g

Snack
Cheesy Baked Eggs
Preparation Time: 5 minutes
Cooking Time: 15 minutes

Servings: 1

Ingredients:

1 tsp., softened butter

2 tsp., milk

2 large eggs

1 tsp. Pepper

1 tsp. salt

2 tablespoon cheddar cheese, shredded

1 tablespoon parmesan cheese, grated

Direction:

Preheat your oven to 400F.

In the meantime, coat inside of an oven ramekin, 8-ounces, with butter.

Whisk milk and eggs in a bowl, small.

Stir in pepper, salt, and cheeses.

Pour the batter into the ramekin.

For about 15-18 minutes, bake until eggs are cooked through.

Enjoy!

Nutrition: calories 350, fat 28g, fiber 1g, carbs 8g, protein 22g

Lunch:
Mashed Cauliflower

Preparation time: 10 minutes
Cooking time: 20 minutes
Servings: 4
Ingredients:
- 1 cup water
- 8 cups cauliflower, sliced into florets
- 2 tbsp. sour cream
- 2 tbsp. heavy cream
- 1 tbsp. butter
- Salt to taste

Directions:
1. Add the water to the Instant Pot.
2. Place the steamer basket inside.
3. Put the cauliflower on top of the basket.
4. Close the pot.
5. Set it to manual.
6. Cook at high pressure for 10 minutes.
7. Puree the cauliflower in the food processor.
8. Stir in the rest of the ingredients

Nutrition: calories 114, fat 7g, fiber 2g, carbs 11g, protein 8g

Dinner:
Ham with BBQ Glaze
Preparation time: 5 minutes
Cooking time: 10 minutes
Servings: 8
Ingredients:
- 1 tbsp. olive oil
- 80 oz. ham slices
- 1 tbsp. chili powder
- 1 tbsp. paprika
- 1 tsp. cumin
- ½ tsp. cinnamon
- ¼ tsp. ground cloves
- 1 tbsp. sucralose sweetener
- 5 tbsp. sugar free apricot preserve

Directions:
1. Set the Instant Pot to sauté.
2. Add the olive oil.
3. Add the ham and cook for 2 to 3 minutes.
4. Remove and set aside.
5. In a bowl, mix the rest of the ingredients.
6. Pour into the pot.
7. Simmer for 1 minute.
8. Toss the ham slices in the mixture before serving.

Nutrition: calories 450, fat 26g, fiber 2g, carbs 4g, protein 6g

Day 18

Breakfast:

Denver Omelet

Preparation time: 4 minutes
Cooking time: 1 minutes
Servings: 1
Ingredients:

- 2 tbsp. butter
- ¼ cup onions, chopped
- ¼ cup green bell pepper, diced
- 2 eggs
- ¼ cup ham, chopped

Directions:

1. Sautee the onions and bell pepper, with the butter, in a small skillet.
2. Whip the eggs and mix the ingredients in a bowl.
3. Microwave for one minute.
4. Pre-cook the peppers and onions and place in zip-lock freezer bags by portions, add the ham to the bags. Freeze. The night before making, place the peppers mix in the fridge to thaw or microwave for one minute before adding to the whipped egg to make.

Nutrition: calories 605, fat 23g, fiber 2g, carbs 8g, protein 2g

Snack
Chocolate Frosty

Preparation time: 3 minutes
Cooking time: 0 minutes
Servings: 1
Ingredients:
- 2 tbsp. chocolate milk
- 2 tbsp. heavy cream
- 2 tbsp. sugar-free chocolate syrup
- ½ cup ice cubes

Directions:
1. In a blender, combine the heavy cream, chocolate syrup, ice cubes. Blend until thick and smooth. Add a bit of chocolate milk for less thick consistency. Add more ice for a thicker consistency.

Nutrition: calories 200, fat 8g, fiber 2g, carbs 8g, protein 6g

Lunch:
Bok Choy with Peanuts
Preparation time: 10 minutes
Cooking time: 10 minutes
Servings: 4
Ingredients:
- 1 oz. water
- 1 packet Splenda
- 2 tbsp. tamari
- 1 tbsp. vegetable oil
- 1 tsp. sesame oil
- 1 tsp. garlic, minced
- 4 green onions, chopped
- 10 cups Chinese cabbage, chopped
- Pinch red pepper flakes
- ¼ cup roasted peanuts

Directions:
1. In a bowl, mix the water, Splenda and tamari.
2. Set the Instant Pot to sauté.
3. Add the oils.
4. Add the garlic, green onion, cabbage and pepper flakes.
5. Pour in the tamari mixture.
6. Cook for 3 minutes, stirring frequently.
7. Top with the peanuts and serve.

Nutrition: calories 125, fat 9g, fiber 2g, carbs 8g, protein 6g

Dinner:
Almond Thin and Crispy Pizza Crust

Preparation time: 30 minutes
Cooking time: 50 minutes
Servings: 2
Ingredients:

- ½ cup Tap Water
- 1 tbsp. Extra Virgin Olive Oil
- 1 ½ cups Almond Meal Flour
- 3 tbsp. Potato Starch
- 1 tsp. Baking Powder
- 1/2 tsp. garlic powder
- ¼ tsp. Salt
- ½ tsp. Xylitol
- ¾ tsp. leaf Oregano
- ¾ tsp. leaf Basil
- 3 servings Organic 100% Whole Ground Golden Flaxseed Meal
- ¼ tsp. Crushed Red Pepper Flakes - 5 tbsp. Flax seeds

Directions:

This formula makes an awesome covering. It is viewed as a Phase 4 formula because of the potato starch despite the fact that it is a low sum.

The potato starch enables the batter to extend somewhat more and to turn out to be increasingly fresh.

1. Whisk together the water and oil in a little bowl. Put aside.
2. Consolidate the staying dry fixings; mixing to mix. The flavors are discretionary yet include a pleasant flavor. Consider signifying 1/2 tsp. garlic powder too.
3. Prepare at 375°F for 20-25 minutes until brilliant and fresh around the edges. Permit to cool around 20 minutes to frame a crunchy outside layer.
4. Top with fixings and spot back in the stove or oven for a couple of minutes to cook the garnishes.

Nutrition: calories 300, fat 23g, fiber 2g, carbs 8g, protein 16g

Day 19

Breakfast:
Atkins Pancakes

Preparation time: 10 minutes
Cooking time: 30 minutes
Servings: 4
Ingredients:

- 4 oz. Vanilla Whey Protein
- ¼ cup Blanched Almond Flour
- ¼ cup Whole Grain Soy Flour
- 1 tsp. Baking Powder
- ½ tsp. Pumpkin Pie Spice
- 4 large Eggs
- ¼ cup Large or Small Curd Creamed Cottage Cheese
- ½ cup Pumpkin

Directions:

1. Make certain to utilize canned pumpkin purée, not pumpkin pie blend (which has included sugar), to make these flapjacks. Present with sans sugar flapjack syrup or almond margarine.
2. Blend the protein powder, almond supper, soy flour, preparing powder and pumpkin pie zest blend in a medium blending bowl. Mix in the beaten eggs, curds, and pumpkin purée until mixed.
3. Make use around 1/4 cup for each hotcake, drop player onto the skillet. At the point when air pockets start to shape in the flapjacks, turn and cook an additional 2 minutes or until firm.
4. Rehash, keeping flapjacks warm in the broiler before serving

Nutrition: calories 123, fat 8g, fiber 2g, carbs 8g, protein 7g

Snack

Ginger Flan

Preparation time: 30 minutes
Cooking time: 20 minutes
Servings: 6
Ingredients:

- 3 egg yolks
- 2 egg
- 1½ cups heavy cream
- 1 cup tap water
- 8 packets sucralose based sweetener
- 1 tsp. pure vanilla extract
- 3 tsp. ground ginger

Directions:

1. Preheat oven to 350°F
2. Place a roasting pan on center shelf of oven. Fill to half with boiling water.
3. In a blender, combine the eggs, egg yolks, water, cream, sugar substitute, ginger, and vanilla. Blend until smooth.
4. Pass the sauce through a sieve. Pour into a 1-quart shallow baking dish.
5. Place the dish in the water bath in the oven. Bake 30-35 minutes.
6. Transfer to a cooling rack.
7. Once cooled, spray plastic wrap with non-stick cooking spray. Place it gently against the flan. Chill in the fridge 3 hours.
8. Once chilled, invert the baking dish and tap the flan onto a serving platter.

Nutrition: calories 265, fat 26g, fiber 0g, carbs 3g, protein 5g

Lunch:
Rosemary Chicken
Preparation time: 30 minutes
Cooking time: 20 minutes
Servings: 2
Ingredients:

- 20 oz. chicken thigh
- 1 tsp. rosemary
- Salt and pepper to taste
- 3 tbsp. olive oil
- 1 cup chicken broth
- 4 oz. white wine
- ½ cup onion, chopped
- 8 oz. mushroom

Directions:
1. Season the chicken with rosemary, salt and pepper.
2. Add the olive oil to the Instant Pot.
3. Set it to sauté.
4. Add the onion and mushroom and cook for 1 minute.
5. Take out of the pot and set aside.
6. Add the chicken and cook until brown on both sides.
7. Pour in the chicken broth and white wine, and toss to coat evenly.
8. Close the pot and choose manual.
9. Cook at high pressure for 5 minutes.
10. Release the pressure naturally.
11. Take the chicken out and set aside.
12. Drizzle the cooking liquid and top the chicken with the onion and mushrooms before serving.

Nutrition: calories 235, fat 26g, fiber 2g, carbs 2g, protein 4g

Dinner:
Almond Muffin in a Mug Recipe

Preparation time: 30 minutes
Cooking time: 35 minutes
Servings: 6
Ingredients:

- ¼ cup Bob's Red Mill Almond Meal
- 1 tsp. No Calorie Sweetener
- ¼ tsp. Baking Powder
- 1 dash Salt
- ½ tsp. Cinnamon
- 1 large Egg
- 1 tsp. Canola Vegetable Oil

Directions:
1. Spot every single dry fixing in an espresso cup. Blend to consolidate.
2. Include the egg and oil. Mix until completely consolidated.
3. Microwave for 1 minute. Utilize a blade if important to help expel the biscuit from the glass, cut, spread, and eat.

Nutrition: calories 200, fat 8g, fiber 2g, carbs 8g, protein 6g

Day 20

Breakfast:
Pumpkin Almond Pancakes

Preparation Time: 5 minutes
Cooking Time: 10 minutes
Servings: 6
Ingredients:

- 4 oz. vanilla whey protein powder
- ½ cup pumpkin puree, canned
- 4 eggs, beaten
- 1 tsp. double acting baking powder, sodium aluminum sulphate
- 1 cup cottage cheese, creamed
- ¼ cup almond flour, blanched
- ½ tsp. pumpkin pie spice
- ¼ cup whole grain soy flour, dry

Directions:
1. Combine the protein powder, pumpkin pie spice, almond flour, baking powder and soy flour together in a bowl.
2. Add the remaining ingredients and mix until well blended.
3. Grease a skillet using butter.
4. Pour ¼ cup of the batter into the skillet and cook over medium heat. Once bubbles form in the middle, flip the pancakes over and cook until firm.
5. Repeat the procedure with the remaining batter.

Nutrition: calories 183, fat 8g, fiber 2g, carbs 4g, protein 21g

Snack
Coconut Cashew Bars
Preparation time: 30 minutes
Cooking time: 20 minutes
Servings: 8
Ingredients:

- 1 cup almond flour
- 1 tsp. cinnamon
- Pinch salt
- ½ cup cashew nuts
- ¼ cup coconut, shredded
- ¼ cup butter, melted
- ¼ cup sugar-free maple syrup

Directions:
1. In a large bowl, combine the flour, cinnamon, salt. Whisk briefly.
2. Smash the cashews. Add them with the coconut to the bowl.
3. Stir in the butter and maple syrup.
4. Line an 8x8 baking dish with parchment paper. Pour in the batter. Spread into an even layer.
5. Place in refrigerator. Chill 2 hours. Slice into bars.

Nutrition: calories 189, fat 18g, fiber 2g, carbs 8g, protein 4g

Lunch:
Chicken Parmesan

Preparation time: 10 minutes
Cooking time: 20 minutes
Servings: 4
Ingredients:

- Salt and pepper to taste
- ¾ serving Atkins flour mix
- 1 egg
- 32 oz. chicken breast fillet, sliced into strips
- 3 tbsp. olive oil
- 2 tbsp. heavy cream
- 1 ¾ cup mozzarella cheese, shredded
- ½ cup Parmesan cheese, grated
- 3 tbsp. basil
- 3 cups tomato sauce

Directions:
1. In the first bowl, combine the salt, pepper and flour.
2. In the second bowl, beat the egg.
3. Dip the chicken strips in the first bowl and then in the second.
4. Heat the oil in the Instant Pot by choosing sauté mode.
5. Cook the chicken until golden brown on both sides.
6. Spread the heavy cream on top of the chicken.
7. Add a layer of tomato sauce.
8. Top with the cheese and basil.
9. Cover the pot.
10. Set it to manual and cook at high pressure for 1 minute.

Nutrition: calories 200, fat 8g, fiber 2g, carbs 8g, protein 6g

Dinner:

Beef Burger with Feta

Preparation time: 15 minutes
Cooking time: 30 minutes
Servings: 4
Ingredients:

- 1 lb. lean ground beef
- 1 spring onion
- ½ cup baby spinach, chopped
- ¼ cup tomato, chopped
- ¼ cup feta cheese, crumbled
- ½ tsp. dill weed, dried
- Salt and pepper to taste
- 1 cup water

Directions:
1. Combine all the ingredients in a large bowl.
2. Form four patties.
3. Wrap each patty with foil.
4. Place the steamer rack inside the pot.
5. Put the wrapped patty on top of the rack.
6. Pour the water into the bottom of the Instant Pot.
7. Cover the pot and select manual mode.
8. Cook at high pressure for 12 minutes.
9. Release the pressure naturally.

Nutrition: calories 200, fat 8g fiber 2g, carbs 8g, protein 6g

Day 21

Breakfast:

Candied Sweet Potatoes

Preparation Time: 20 minutes
Cooking Time: 40 minutes
Servings: 6
Ingredients:

- ½ cup maple flavored syrup, sugar free
- 3 tbsp. butter, unsalted
- 3 tsp. ginger
- 4 sweet potato, baked

Directions:

1. Preheat oven to 450°F. Grease an 8" by 10" baking dish using butter.
2. Let the salted water boil and cook sweet potatoes in it for about 8-10 minutes. Drain excess water.
3. Cook ginger and syrup together over low heat for about 3 minutes.
4. Place the sweet potatoes in a single layer on the prepared baking dish and drizzle the syrup mixture over them.
5. Cover the baking dish with aluminum foil and place it in the oven. Cook for about 40 minutes.

Nutrition: calories 133, fat 8g, fiber 2g, carbs 8g, protein 6g

Snack

Choco Peanut Tart

Preparation time: 30 minutes
Cooking time: 20 minutes
Servings: 4
Ingredients:
Crust:
- ¼ cup flaxseed
- 2 tbsp. almond flour
- 1 tbsp. Erythritol
- 1 large egg (just need the egg white)

Middle Layer:
- 4 tbsp. smooth peanut butter
- 2 tbsp. unsalted butter

Top Layer:
- 1 medium avocado
- 4 tbsp. cocoa powder
- ¼ cup Erythritol
- ½ tsp. pure vanilla extract
- ½ tsp. cinnamon - 2 tbsp. heavy cream

Directions:
1. Preheat oven to 350°F Whisk the egg white. In a large bowl, grind the flaxseed to a powdery consistency.
2. Add the almond flour, Erythritol. Stir in the egg white until crumbly.
3. Pour the mixture into a pie dish. Press in an even layer along bottom of pie dish. Bake for 8 minutes. Cool the crust completely before filling.
4. In a separate bowl, mash the avocado until smooth. Add the cocoa powder, Erythritol, cinnamon, vanilla extract, cream. Whisk until smooth.
5. In a separate bowl, melt the butter. Add peanut butter. Stir until smooth.
6. Pour the peanut butter batter in the pie dish. Spread in an even layer.
7. Pour the chocolate layer over the peanut butter layer. Smooth it out.

Nutrition: calories 123, fat 8g, fiber 2g, carbs 8g, protein 7g

Lunch:
Steamed Mussels in coconut Broth

Preparation Time: 10 Minutes
Cooking Time: 15 Minutes
Servings: 4
Ingredients:
- 2 tbsp. butter
- 1 cup shallots, chopped
- 2 cloves garlic, minced
- 2 tsp. Italian seasoning
- 3 tsp. stevia
- 10 oz. bottle of clam juice
- 1 cup cherry tomatoes
- 2 lbs. mussels, cleaned and washed

Finishing Ingredients:
- 1 cup coconut milk
- 1 tsp. tapioca starch

Directions:
1. Using the sauté mode, melt the butter in the Instant Pot.
2. Add the shallots and cook until soft (approximately 2 minutes,)
3. Add the garlic and cook until aromatic (approximately 1 minute.)
4. Stir in the cherry tomatoes, increase the heat until the mixture starts to boil.
5. Add the rest of the Ingredients (except finishing Ingredients) and return to a boil.
6. Stir in the mussels until everything is combined.
7. Close the lid and lock it.
8. Set the vent to Sealing.
9. Cook on high pressure for 6 minutes.
10. When the timer beeps, quickly release the steam.
11. Serve.

Nutrition: calories 200, fat 8g, fiber 2g, carbs 8g, protein 6g

Dinner:
Instant Pot Crab Bisque
Preparation Time: 10 Minutes
Cooking Time: 22 Minutes
Servings: 8
Ingredients:
- 2 lbs. crab meat
- 2 cups seafood broth
- 2 onions, chopped
- A stalk celery, chopped
- 1 tablespoon minced Garlic
- 2 medium sized Carrots
- 1 large Bell pepper
- 1/2 cup tomatoes, crushed
- 4 tsp. tomato paste
- 4 tbsp. butter
- 1 tsp. avocado oil
- 1/2 cup cream
- 2 bay leaves

Herbs & Spices Ingredients:
- 2 tsp old bay seasoning
- 1 tsp. dry thyme
- ¼ tsp. smoked paprika
- Salt and black pepper, to taste

Topping Ingredients:
- 2 tomato, chopped
- 1 stalks cilantro, chopped
- 2 tsp. olive oil
- 1/2 tsp. dry thyme
- 1 tsp. chili flakes

Directions.

1. Combine the topping Ingredients; set aside.
2. Put the butter, oil, and bay leaf in the Instant Pot; using the sauté mode, melt the butter.
3. Add the onions and cook for 2 minutes.
4. Add the garlic; cook for 1 minute (until aromatic.)
5. Stir in the herbs and seasoning Ingredients, celery, carrots, and bell pepper; cook 2-3 minutes.
6. Add the tomatoes, crab meat, tomato paste, and broth.
7. Close the lid and lock it.
8. Set the vent to Sealing.
9. Cook on high for 12-15 minutes.
10. When the timer beeps, naturally release the steam.
11. Open the lid.
12. Now mix in the cream, stirring well.
13. Mix with an immersion blender or transfer to a regular blender; blend until smooth.
14. Pour into individual bowls.
15. Serve with topping.

Nutrition: calories 256, fat 8g, fiber 2g, carbs 16g, protein 23g

XHAΠTEP 7:

Meal Plan Day 22-28

Day 22

Breakfast:
Strawberry Smoothie Bowl
Preparation time: 30 minutes
Cooking time: 0 minutes
Servings: 2
Ingredients:
Smoothie bowl:

- 1½ cups frozen strawberries
- ½ cup coconut milk
- 1 cup ,Chia seeds
- 6 Strawberries
- 2 Banana

Directions:

1. In a blender jug, puree all the ingredients for the smooth bowl.
2. Pour the smoothie in the serving bowl.
3. Add strawberries, banana and chia seeds on top.
4. Chill well then serve.

Nutrition: calories 210, fat 14g, fiber 5g, carbs 8g, protein 3g

Snack
Mini Vanilla Cloud Cupcakes
Preparation time: 10 minutes
Cooking time: 20 minutes
Servings: 8
Ingredients:
Cupcakes:
- 6 large eggs, room temperature
- 6 tbsp. cream cheese, room temperature
- ½ tsp. cream of tartar
- 2 tsp. pure vanilla extract
- ¼ cup granulated stevia/Erythritol mixture

Frosting:
1. ½ cup cream cheese, room temperature
2. 2 tbsp. butter, room temperature
3. ⅓ cup granulated stevia/Erythritol mix
4. 1 tbsp. pure vanilla extract

Directions:
1. Preheat oven to 300°F
2. Separate the eggs yolks and egg whites.
3. Spray 2 muffin tins with non-stick cooking spray.
4. In a bowl, using an electric mixer, beat the cream cheese until smooth. Add the egg yolks one at a time. Stir in sweetener and vanilla extract until smooth batter.
5. In a separate bowl, whip egg whites until fluffy. Stir in cream of tartar.
6. Combine the egg whites with the egg yolk batter. Fold in gently until combined.
7. Using an ice cream scoop, fill the muffin tin cups ¾ full.
8. Place tin in oven. Bake 30-35 minutes, until toothpick comes out dry.
9. Place on cooling rack. Cool completely before icing.
10. In a bowl, combine the cream cheese and butter. Whip with electric mixer until smooth. Add the sweetener and vanilla. Whip until smooth.

Nutrition: calories 200, fat 8g, fiber 2g, carbs 8g, protein 6g

Lunch:
Sautéed Beef with Veggies
Preparation time: 10 minutes
Cooking time: 30 minutes
Servings: 4
Ingredients:
- 1 tbsp. olive oil
- 1 ½ lb. lean ground beef
- ¼ cup onion, chopped
- ¼ cup bell pepper, chopped
- 15 oz. tomato sauce
- 4 tbsp. tomato paste
- Salt and pepper to taste
- 6 cups Romaine lettuce, shredded
- 6 oz. cheddar cheese, shredded

Directions:
1. Pour the olive oil into the Instant Pot.
2. Add the onion and peppers.
3. Cook for 1 minute.
4. Add the beef and cook until brown.
5. Drain the excess fat.
6. Pour in the tomato sauce and paste.
7. Season with the salt and pepper.
8. Cover the pot.
9. Set it to manual.
10. Cook at high pressure for 5 minutes.
11. Release the pressure naturally.
12. Serve on top of shredded Romaine, and sprinkle cheese on top.

Nutrition: calories 575, fat 28g, fiber 2g, carbs 3g, protein 64g

Dinner:
Blackened Salmon
Preparation time: 10 minutes
Cooking time: 20 minutes
Servings: 4
Ingredients:
- 3 tsp. leaves oregano
- 3 tsp. thyme
- 1 tbsp. old bay seasoning
- Salt and pepper to taste
- ¼ cup vegetable oil
- 24 oz. salmon fillets

Directions:
1. Combine the oregano, thyme, old bay seasoning, salt and pepper in a bowl.
2. Coat the fish with oil and sprinkle the herb mixture generously on both sides of the fish.
3. Heat the remaining oil in the Instant Pot by pressing the sauté function.
4. Cook the salmon until the coating is black or about 3 minutes on each side

Nutrition: calories 345, fat 24g, fiber 2g, carbs 8g, protein 33g

Day 23

Breakfast:
Belgian Waffles Recipe

Preparation time: 10 minutes
Cooking time: 30 minutes
Servings: 4
Ingredients:

- 1 cup Whole Grain Soy Flour
- 2 tbsp. Sucralose Based Sweetener
- 3 tsp. Baking Powder
- 1/2 tsp. salt
- 1/4 cup Heavy Cream
- 3 large Eggs
- 1 tbsp. Sugar-Free Syrup
- 1/4 cup Water

Directions:

1. Heat waffle iron per maker's guidelines.
2. Whisk together soy flour, sugar substitute, preparing powder and salt. Include cream, eggs and syrup and mix until very much mixed. Include cold water 1 tablespoon at once until batter is effectively spreadable, about the consistency of a thick hotcake batter.
3. Shower waffle iron with oil splash. Spot around 3 tablespoons of batter in the middle of a waffle iron. Cook as indicated by producer's directions until fresh and dim brilliant darker. Repeat with the rest of the batter. Serve warm.

Nutrition: calories 115, fat 8g, fiber 2g, carbs 5g, protein 9g

Snack
Pumpkin Pecan Pie Ice Cream
Preparation time: 10 minutes
Cooking time: 20 minutes
Servings: 4
Ingredients:
- ½ cup cottage cheese
- ½ cup pumpkin puree
- 2 cups coconut milk
- 3 large egg yolks
- ½ tsp. Xanthan gum
- 20 drops liquid Stevia
- 1 tsp. pure maple extract
- 1 tsp. pumpkin spice
- ½ cup toasted pecans, chopped
- 2 tbsp. salted butter

Directions:
1. In a skillet, melt some butter. Toast the pecans. Set aside to cool.
2. In a separate bowl, combine the cottage cheese, pumpkin puree, coconut milk, egg yolks. Blend with electric mixer.
3. Stir in toasted pecans, xanthan gum, pumpkin spice, liquid stevia, maple extract.
4. Pour the mixture into an ice cream machine.
5. Churn according to instruction of ice cream machine. Serve.

Nutrition: calories 260, fat 22g, fiber 2g, carbs 8g, protein 6g

Lunch:
Snapper in Lemon Wine Sauce
Preparation time: 10 minutes
Cooking time: 40 minutes
Servings: 6
Ingredients:
- ¼ cup olive oil
- 1 tsp. salt
- ¼ tsp. black pepper
- 1 tsp. paprika
- ¼ cup lemon juice
- 4 oz. sauvignon blanc wine
- ¼ cup parsley
- 8 tbsp. basil
- 6 lb. snapper
- Cooking spray

Directions:
1. In a bowl, mix the oil, salt, pepper and paprika.
2. Pour in the lemon juice and wine.
3. Add the parsley and basil.
4. Marinate the fish in half of this mixture for 30 minutes.
5. Spray the Instant Pot with oil.
6. Switch it to sauté.
7. Brown the fish on both sides.
8. Add the remaining mixture.
9. Cover the pot and set it to manual.
10. Cook at high pressure for 3 minutes.
11. Release the pressure quickly.

Nutrition: calories 311, fat 8g, fiber 2g, carbs 2g, protein 45g

Dinner:
Spicy Tofu with Tamarind Sauce
Preparation time: 10 minutes
Cooking time: 20 minutes
Servings: 4
Ingredients:
- 28 oz. firm tofu, sliced
- 3 tbsp. olive oil
- Salt and pepper to taste
- 1 tbsp. tamarinds, pulp
- ¼ cup water
- 3 tsp. garlic, minced
- 1 tbsp. shallots, chopped
- ¼ tbsp. red chili paste
- 2 oz. dry roasted peanuts
- 2 tbsp. creamy peanut butter
- ¼ cup coconut milk

Directions:
1. Rub tofu with half of the oil.
2. Season with the salt and pepper.
3. Dissolve the tamarind in water.
4. Set the Instant Pot to sauté.
5. Pour in the remaining oil.
6. Cook the garlic and shallots for 1 minute.
7. Add the chili paste, peanuts, peanut butter, tamarind juice, coconut milk.
8. Mix well.
9. Add the tofu.
10. Press the sauté setting to thicken the sauce.
11. Drizzle the sauce over the tofu before serving.

Nutrition: calories 422, fat 33g, fiber 2g, carbs 3g, protein 6g

Day 24

Breakfast:

Cinnamon Chocolate Smoothie

Preparation time: 4 minutes
Cooking time: 0 minutes
Servings: 1
Ingredients:

- ½ cup firm Tofu
- 2 tbsp. cocoa powder
- 1 scoop chocolate protein powder
- 2 tbsp. cinnamon
- 2 sweetener packets
- 1 cup almond milk, unsweetened
- 4 ice cubes

Directions:

1. Place all the ingredients in a blender, pulse until desired consistency, and serve.
2. Refrigerate the tofu. Place all the dry ingredients into one snack sized zip-lock bag.

Nutrition: calories 273, fat 13g, fiber 2g, carbs 8g, protein 5g

Snack
Amaretti Cookies
Preparation time: 10 minutes
Cooking time: 20 minutes
Servings: 4
Ingredients:
- 1 cup almond flour
- 2 tbsp. coconut flour
- ½ tsp. baking powder
- ¼ tsp. cinnamon
- ½ tsp. salt
- ½ cup Erythritol
- 1 tbsp. shredded coconut
- 4 tbsp. coconut oil
- 2 large eggs
- ½ tsp. pure vanilla extract
- 1 cup, Shredded Coconut
- 2 tbsp. sugar-free jam

Directions:
1. Preheat oven to 350°F
2. Line a cookie sheet with parchment paper.
3. In a bowl, combine the almond flour, coconut flour, baking powder, cinnamon, salt, Erythritol. Whisk together.
4. In another bowl, add the coconut oil. Stir to soften it. Stir in one egg at a time. Add the vanilla. Stir until combined.
5. Add dry ingredients to wet ingredients. Stir until just combined.
6. Using a tablespoon, scoop cookie dough onto cookie sheet; 1 inch apart.
7. Dab your finger in water, and press an indent in the middle of the dough.
8. Bake 16 minutes.
9. Place on a cooling rack. Cool 30 minutes.
10. Add 1 teaspoon of jam to indent in cookie. Garnish with shredded coconut.

Nutrition: calories 85, fat 8g, fiber 1g, carbs 3g, protein 3g

Lunch:
Spaghetti Squash with Tomato Pesto
Preparation time: 10 minutes
Cooking time: 30 minutes
Servings: 4
Ingredients:
- 1 spaghetti squash, sliced in half and seeds removed
- 1 cup water
- 1 tbsp. olive oil
- 4 oz. firm tofu, sliced into cubes
- 3 cups sugar free tomato pesto sauce

Directions:
1. Place the steamer basket inside the Instant Pot.
2. Add the water.
3. Put the squash on top of the basket.
4. Secure the pot.
5. Select manual setting.
6. Cook at high pressure for 7 minutes.
7. Release the pressure quickly.
8. Use a fork to separate the strands of the squash.
9. Drain the water from the pot.
10. Fry the tofu until golden.
11. Toss the spaghetti strands with tomato pesto sauce and top with the tofu.

Nutrition: calories 128, fat 6g, fiber 2g, carbs 18g, protein 3g

Dinner:
Cauliflower & Green Beans with Oyster Sauce

Preparation time: 10 minutes
Cooking time: 20 minutes
Servings: 4
Ingredients:

- 1 cup water
- 1 ¼ lb. cauliflower, sliced into florets
- 4 oz. green beans
- 2 tbsp. vegetable oil
- 2 tsp. ginger
- 1 clove garlic
- 3 green onions
- 2 tbsp. oyster sauce
- 2 tbsp. tamari
- 1 tsp. sucralose sweetener
- 1/8 cup almonds, slivered

Directions:

1. Add a cup of water to the Instant Pot.
2. Place the steamer rack inside.
3. Add the cauliflower and green beans.
4. Cover the pot. Set it to manual function.
5. Cook at high pressure for 3 minutes. Release the pressure quickly.
6. Drain the water. Set aside the vegetables.
7. Pour the oil into the pot.
8. Switch it to sauté.
9. Add the garlic, ginger and onions.
10. Put the vegetables back to the pot.
11. Mix the oyster sauce, tamari and sweetener.
12. Simmer for 5 minutes. Sprinkle almonds on top.

Nutrition: calories 130, fat 8g, fiber 5g, carbs 12g, protein 32g

Day 25

Breakfast:
Eggs, Ham, and Spinach Pancakes

Preparation Time: 5 Minutes
Cooking Time: 10 Minutes
Servings: 4
Ingredients:
- 2 yellow onions, diced
- 3 cups ham, chopped
- 3 cups baby spinach, chopped
- 2 slices cheddar cheese, shredded
- 2 tbsp. Parmesan cheese
- 8 large eggs
- ½ cup almond milk, unsweetened
- Salt and freshly ground black pepper to taste
- Oil spray for greasing

Directions:
1. Coat the inside of an Instant Pot with cooking spray.
2. Whisk the eggs in a bowl.
3. Add in the ham, onions, spinach, cheeses, salt, and pepper; mix thoroughly
4. Add the almond milk; stir to mix in.
5. Pour the mixture into the Instant Pot.
6. Lock the lid to the Instant Pot.
7. Cook for 10 minutes on high pressure.
8. Turn the Instant Pot off when the timer beeps; after a minute quick release the steam.
9. Remove the top from the Instant Pot.
10. Loosen the pancake from the sides and bottom of the Instant Pot.
11. Transfer the pancake to a plate.
12. Serve the pancake with your chosen topping

Nutrition: calories 473, fat 8g, fiber 2g, carbs 8g, protein 39g

Snack
Beet-Pickled Deviled Eggs

Preparation Time: 10 minutes
Cooking Time: 20 minutes
Servings: 12 pieces
Ingredients:
- 6 large eggs
- 1 cup apple cider vinegar
- 16 oz. jar pickled beets
- ⅓ Cup brown sugar
- 1 tbsp. whole peppercorns
- 1 tsp. salt
- Fresh rosemary leaves, chopped

Directions:
1. Hard boil the eggs and then let them cool. Peel off the shells and set aside.
2. Pour the jar of beets into a large bowl, then add apple cider vinegar, peppercorns, sugar, and salt. Stir to combine well. This is your brine.
3. Carefully place peeled eggs into the brine and refrigerate for at least 12 hours. No more than 3 days in the brine.
4. Remove from the brine solution and cut each egg in half, top to bottom. Scoop out the yolk of each egg carefully and place it in a bowl. Mash all the egg yolk.
5. Take the egg yolk mixture and distribute evenly between all of the formed egg whites using a spoon.
6. Garnish with the chopped rosemary and they are ready to serve. This is a great snack.

Nutrition: calories 178, fat 8g, fiber 2g, carbs 18g, protein 3g

Lunch:
Buffalo Wings
Preparation time: 10 minutes
Cooking time: 40 minutes
Servings: 6
Ingredients:
For marinate
- 1 egg, beaten
- 32 oz. chicken wings
- 1 cup vinegar
- Salt and pepper to taste
- ½ cup vegetable oil
- ½ tsp. garlic powder
- ¼ tsp. celery salt
- 1/8 tsp cayenne pepper

For dressing
- 16 tbsp. mayonnaise
- ½ cup cultured sour cream
- 1 green onion
- ¼ cup blue cheese
- 1 tbsp. lemon juice - 1 clove garlic, crushed

Directions:
1. Mix the marinade ingredients in a large bowl.
2. Add the egg into the bowl. Take a few tablespoons of the marinade and drizzle all over the chicken. Marinate for 30 minutes.
3. Pour the rest into the Instant Pot. Close the pot. Choose manual mode.
4. Cook at high pressure for 5 minutes. Release the pressure quickly. Drain the liquid. Pour the olive oil into the Instant Pot. Switch to sauté.
5. Cook until the chicken is slightly fried.
6. Mix the ingredients for the dressing.
7. Serve the chicken wings with the dressing.

Nutrition: calories 640, fat 44g, fiber 1g, carbs 8g, protein 46g

Dinner:

Vegetarian Poke Bowl

Preparation time: 10 Minutes
Cooking time: 35 Minutes
Serving: 2
Ingredients:

- 200g sushi or jasmine rice
- 12 small carrots
- 1.2 Hokkaido or butternut squash
- 2 tsp. olive oil
- 1 slice ,pineapple
- 3 tsp., Kikkoman poke sauce
- 50 g sprouts
- 2-3 handful corn salad
- 1 cup pumpkin seeds
- Handful ,Fresh mint

Directions:

1. Cook sushi or jasmine rice according to the package directions. Allow to cool slightly, and then spread on 4 bowls.
2. Dice the pumpkin and then place it inside a casserole dish with the whole carrots. Sprinkle with olive oil, season it with salt, season with pepper and bake at 180°C for 30 minutes. After the baking, mix with kikkoman poke sauce and Hokkaido or butternut squash, pumpkin seeds.
3. Pcel and dice the pineapple.
4. Add pineapple, sprouts, and heifer seedlings; add corn salad, carrots and pumpkin to each bowl. Garnish with some fresh mint and additionally serve kikkoman poke sauce as a side dish.

Nutrition: calories 200, fat 8g, fiber 2g, carbs 8g, protein 6g

Day 26

Breakfast:

Spinach, Goat Cheese and Chorizo Omelet

Preparation Time: 15 Minutes
Cooking Time: 12-15 Minutes
Servings: 3
Ingredients:

- 3 oz. chorizo sausage
- 1/3 tbsp. butter
- 3 eggs
- 1 tbsp. water
- 1 oz. fresh goat cheese, crumbled
- ½ cup baby spinach leaves
- 3 avocados, sliced and optional

Directions:

1. Remove the casing from the chorizo and place it in a medium frying pan; cook thoroughly, breaking it up with a spatula as it cooks.
2. In the meantime, use a small bowl to beat the eggs and water.
3. When completely cooked, removed the chorizo from the frying pan with a slotted spoon and place it on a paper towel.
4. Wipe the pan clean with a different paper towel.
5. Turn the burner temperature to low, and melt the butter.
6. Pour the eggs into the pan.
7. Use the chorizo, spinach and goat cheese to cover half of the eggs.
8. Cover the pan and cook until the eggs are cooked through.
9. If the eggs are browning, turn off the heat to finish cooking. The residual heat will continue to cook the eggs for approximately 10 minutes more.
10. If desired, serve the omelet with avocado slices

Nutrition: calories 624, fat 8g, fiber 2g, carbs 8g, protein 17g

Snack
Baked Tofu with Barbecue Rub
Preparation Time: 40 Minutes
Cooking Time: 30 Minutes
Servings: 2
Ingredients:
- 6 oz tofu, firm silken
- 2 tsp. olive oil
- 1 serving Atkins barbecue rub

Directions:
1. Preheat the oven to 375°F.
2. Drain the tofu and pat it dry with a paper towel.
3. Cut the tofu into ¼-inch strips.
4. Mix the olive oil and barbecue rub; rub the mixture onto the tofu.
5. You may allow the tofu to sit 30 minutes to marinate or cook it immediately.
6. Coat a cookie sheet with cooking spray; spread the tofu strips onto the sheet.
7. Bake the tofu for 15 minutes on one side; turn it over and cook it for an additional 15 minutes on the other side. It should be brown and crispy.
8. Remove from the oven to a plate.

Nutrition: calories 200, fat 8g, fiber 2g, carbs 8g, protein 6g

Lunch:
Pineapple Smoothie
Preparation Time: 5 minutes
Cooking time: 1
Servings: 1
Ingredients:
- ½ cup plain yogurt
- ¼ cup fresh or frozen pineapple pieces
- 20 almonds, blanched
- ½ cup almond milk

Direction:
1. In a blender, combine yogurt, pineapple, almonds, almond milk. Blend until a smooth consistency.
2. You can add ice cubes if you want a cooler smoothie.

Nutrition: calories 280, fat 18g, fiber 2g, carbs 18g, protein 10g

Dinner:
Garlic Feta Asparagus
Preparation Time: 10 minutes
Cooking Time: 15 Minutes
Serving: 2
Ingredients:
- 2 lbs. asparagus, trimmed
- 2 tbsp. fresh parsley, chopped
- 4 oz. feta cheese, crumbled
- ½ tsp. red pepper flakes
- ½ tsp. dried oregano
- 3 garlic cloves, minced
- 1 tsp. lemon zest
- ¼ cup olive oil
- 1 tps[,lemon juice
- 1 tps Pepper
- 1 tps Salt

Directions:
1. In a bowl, whisk together oil, oregano, red pepper flakes, garlic, and lemon zest.
2. Add asparagus, crumbled cheese, pepper, and salt and toss well.
3. Transfer asparagus mixture into the air fryer basket and cook at 350 F for 8 minutes.
4. Drizzle asparagus with lemon juice and sprinkle with parsley.
5. Serve and enjoy.

Nutrition: calories 234, fat 20g, fiber 2g, carbs 11g, protein 9g

Day 27

Breakfast:
Low Carb Waffles
Preparation Time: 10 Minutes
Cooking Time: 4 Minutes
Servings: 2
Ingredients:
- 3 egg whites
- 3 tbsp. coconut flour
- 2 tbsp. unsweetened almond milk
- 1/3 tsp. baking powder
- 2 tbsp. stevia, optional

Directions:
1. Preheat the waffle iron to its highest setting after coating it with nonstick spray.
2. In a mixing bowl, whip the eggs whites into stiff peaks using a hand mixer. Add in the remaining ingredients. Pour the waffle mix into the hot waffle iron.
3. The recipe makes 1-2 waffles, depending on the size of your waffle iron.
4. Cook until browned, approximately 3-4 minutes.
5. Serve the waffle with your favorite low carbs fruits.

Nutrition: calories 200, fat 8g, fiber 2g, carbs 8g, protein 6g

Snack
Atkin Brownies

Preparation Time: 20 Minutes
Cooking Time: 35 Minutes
Servings: 4
Ingredients:
- 6 oz. chocolate squares, dark chocolate and unsweetened
- 1 cup butter stick
- 1 cup heavy cream
- 4 large eggs
- 1 cup stevia
- 2 tsp. baking powder (straight phosphate, double-acting)
- 4 servings Atkin flour mix

Directions:
1. Preheat your oven to 335°F.
2. Using a medium bowl, melt the butter and chocolate in the microwave oven; you may use the stovetop instead and then transfer the mixture to a medium bowl.
3. Stir the mixture to ensure that the chocolate has melted completely.
4. Whisk in the heavy cream.
5. In a mixing bowl, beat together whole eggs and sugar substitute until just blended.
6. Using low speed, dump it into the chocolate mixture.
7. Stir in the Atkin flour mix and baking powder with a spoon.
8. Coat a medium baking pan with cooking spray.
9. Spread the batter into the pan making sure that it is even.
10. Bake for 30-35 minutes.
11. Remove the brownies from the oven and allow them to cool on a cooling rack.
12. When cool, cut into pieces.
13. Remove the cookies to a plate or storage container.

Nutrition: calories 583, fat 57g, fiber 2g, carbs 28g, protein 36g

Lunch:
Herbed Butter Fish with Broccoli

Preparation Time: 20 Minutes
Cooking Time: 35 Minutes
Serving: 6
Ingredients:

- 2 cups water
- 6 oz. fish fillet
- 1 tsp. dried basil, divided
- 1 tsp. dried rosemary, divided
- 1 tsp. dried oregano, divided
- 2 tbsp. butter, divided
- 1 cup broccoli, chopped
- Salt to taste

Directions:

1. Pour the water into the Instant Pot.
2. Add the steamer rack inside.
3. Place the fish fillet on a foil sheet.
4. Put the broccoli on another foil sheet.
5. Season both fish and broccoli with the salt, herbs and butter.
6. Wrap the fish and broccoli with the foil sheets.
7. Place the fish packet on top of the rack.
8. Seal the pot, choose manual setting.
9. Cook at high pressure for 8 minutes.
10. Release the pressure naturally.
11. Place the broccoli packet on the rack.
12. Seal the pot and cook at high pressure for 10 minutes.
13. Release the pressure quickly.
14. Serve fish with the broccoli.

Nutrition: calories 319, fat 22g, fiber 2g, carbs 18g, protein 14g

Dinner:
Healthy Air Fryer Mushrooms
Preparation Time: 10 minutes
Cooking Time: 12 Minutes
Servings: 2
Ingredients:
- 8 oz. mushrooms, sliced
- 1 tbsp. parsley, chopped
- 1 tsp. soy sauce
- 1/2 tsp. garlic powder
- 1 tbsp. olive oil
- Pepper
- Salt

Directions:
1. Add all ingredients into the mixing bowl and toss well.
2. Transfer mushrooms in air fryer basket and cook at 380°F for 10-12 minutes. Shake basket halfway through.
3. Serve and enjoy.

Nutrition: calories 89, fat 6g, fiber 2g, carbs 4g, protein 3g

Day 28

Breakfast:

Green Tea Infused Cantaloupe Soup

Preparation Time: 10 minutes

Cooking Time: 20 minutes

Servings: 4

Ingredients:

- 1 ½ cups cantaloupe
- ½ cup brewed green tea
- 1 tsp. fresh minutest sprigs

Directions:

1. Place in a blender the diced cantaloupe.
2. Blend well until puréed. As the blender is running, gradually add in ½ cup of green tea.
3. Continue blending until smooth and free of lumps.
4. Take a spatula and spoon out the mixture into 4 separate soup bowls.
5. Garnish with minutest sprigs on the side.

Nutrition: calories 61, fat 3g, fiber 2g, carbs 11g, protein 61g

Snack
Atkins Cookies
Preparation Time: 25 Minutes
Cooking Time: 12 Minutes
Servings: 8
Ingredients:
- 2 tsp. baking powder
- Pinch salt
- 1 cup butter stick, unsalted
- ½ cup stevia
- 1 tbsp. vanilla extract
- 2 large eggs
- 4 oz. sugar-free chocolate chips
- 6 servings Atkins flour mix

Directions:
1. Preheat the oven to 375°F.
2. Melt the butter in the microwave oven or a small pan on the stovetop.
3. Mix the dry ingredients (baking powder, salt, and flour mix) in a medium bowl; set aside.
4. Using an electric mixer; stir together the butter, sugar substitute, and vanilla extract.
5. Add the eggs one at a time; mixing into the batter as they are added.
6. Add in the dry ingredients a little at a time.
7. Mix the chocolate chips into the batter using a spatula or wooden spoon.
8. Drop the dough onto the cookie sheet in rounded teaspoonful's; press down gently on the cookies with a spatula or your hand.
9. Cook for 10-12 minutes or until brown.
10. Remove the cookies from the oven and transfer them to a plate or cooling rack.
11. The cookies may be served warm or after they have cooled.

Nutrition: calories 297, fat 8g, fiber 2g, carbs 8g, protein 6g

Lunch:
Pizza Fat Bombs
Preparation time: 10 minutes
Cooking time: 40 minutes
Servings: 6
Ingredients:
- ¼ cup cream cheese
- 12 slices pepperoni
- 6 black olives, pitted
- 2 tbsp. sun dried tomato pesto
- 2 tbsp. fresh basil, chopped
- Pinch salt and pepper

Directions:
1. Dice up the pepperoni. Dice the black olives.
2. In a bowl, combine the cream cheese and tomato pesto. Stir in the pepperoni, black olives, and basil. Mash it all with a fork.
3. Pinch off some mixture, roll into 1 inch balls.
4. Place on a tray. Freeze 20 minutes. Serve.

Nutrition: calories 200, fat 8g, fiber 2g, carbs 8g, protein 6g

Dinner:
Pork Sirloin Steak

Preparation time: 10 minutes
Cooking Time: 15 minutes
Serving: 2
Ingredients:

- 1/2 onion
- 4 slices ginger
- 5 cloves garlic
- 1 tsp. allspice powder
- 1 tsp. fennel, ground
- 1 tsp. cinnamon ground
- 1 tsp. cayenne pepper
- 1 tsp. salt
- 1 lb. boneless pork sirloin steaks

Directions:

1. In a blender, jug add all the ingredients except the chops.
2. Rub the chops with this blended mixture and marinate for 30 minutes.
3. Transfer the chops to the Air fryer basket.
4. Press "Power Button" of Air Fry Oven and turn the dial to select the "Air Fry" mode.
5. Press the Time button and again turn the dial to set the cooking time to 15 minutes.
6. Now push the Temp button and rotate the dial to set the temperature at 330°F.
7. Once preheated, place the Air fryer basket in the oven and close its lid.
8. Flip the chops when cooked halfway through then resume cooking.

Nutrition: calories 453, fat 3g, fiber 2g, carbs 2g, protein 23g

ХНАПТЕР 8:

Meal Plan Day 29-31

Day 29

Breakfast:

Pear and Pecan Salad

Preparation Time: 10 minutes
Cooking Time: 30 minutes
Servings: 6
Ingredients:

- ½ cup Gouda cheese
- ½ cup pecans (halved)
- 1 tbsp. unsalted butter
- 3 tbsp. walnut oil
- 1 medium sized pear (sliced into wedges)
- 1/8 tsp. curry powder
- ¾ tsp. salt
- ¼ tsp. freshly ground black pepper
- 2 tsps. sucralose sweetener
- 10 cups salad leaves (lightly packed)
- 1/8 tsp. red pepper
- ¾ cup white wine vinegar

Directions:

Spiced pecans:

1. In a medium sized non-stick skillet, melt the butter over medium heat.
2. Add in the pecans, 1 tsp. of the sucralose, salt, curry powder, and black pepper.
3. Stir the mixture using a wooden spoon for about 4-5 minutes Utes, or until the pecans are toasted evenly.
4. Make sure that the nuts are coated well with the spices.
5. Set aside in a small bowl to cool.
6. In another bowl mix, pears, gouda cheese, vinegar, red pepper, salad leaves, and olive oil to make the salad.
7. Serve with spiced pecans on the side or placed in an entirely separate bowl.

Nutrition: calories 220, fat 16g, fiber 2g, carbs 8g, protein 1g

Snack
Coconut Muffin
Preparation Time: 10 minutes
Cooking Time: 5 minutes
Servings: 1
Ingredients:
- 1 large egg
- 2 tbsp. almond meal flour
- ½ tsp. cinnamon
- 1 tsp. sucralose based sugar substitute
- 1/3 tbsp. coconut flour (organic & high fiber)
- 1/8 tsp. salt
- ¼ tsp. baking powder
- 1 tsp. extra virgin olive oil

Directions:
1. Add all the dry ingredients in a coffee mug and stir well to combine.
2. Next, add extra virgin oil and the egg to the mixture and stir until thoroughly combined.
3. Microwave the mixture for a minutest! Finally, use a knife to remove the muffin from the cup. Slice it and butter well to eat.

Nutrition: calories 207, fat 18g, fiber 2g, carbs 8g, protein 7g

Lunch:
Satisfying Pork Stew

Preparation time: 10 Minutes
Cooking time: 35 Minutes
Serving: 2
Ingredients:
- 1 small onion, thinly sliced
- ½ small cabbage, cut into 4 wedges
- 3 cloves of garlic, smashed
- ¼ lb. baby carrots
- 1 ½ lb. pork shoulder, cut into 1-inch cubes
- ½ tbsp. your favorite seasoning blend
- ½ tbsp. fish sauce
- ½ low-carb marinara sauce
- ½ tbsp. vinegar
- Salt and pepper to taste

Directions:
1. Slice the carrots, onions and garlic, and place in the cooker.
2. Season the beef with your favorite seasoning and layer the pork cubes over the vegetables in the slow cooker.
3. Add the cabbage wedges and top with the marinara sauce
4. Let cook 8-10 hours on Low.
5. Season with salt, pepper, vinegar and herbs before serving.

Nutrition: calories 270, fat 7g, fiber 2g, carbs 8g, protein 24g

Dinner:
Light Mushroom Risotto

Preparation time: 10 Minutes
Cooking time: 35 Minutes
Serving: 2
Ingredients:

- 5 medium potatoes
- 300 g mushrooms
- 250 g arborous rice or carnaroli
- 1 onion
- 1 clove garlic
- 1 l vegetable broth
- 1 glass white wine
- 50 g Parmesan cheese
- 4 tbsp. olive oil
- A sprig parsley
- Salt and pepper

Directions:

1. Heat the vegetable broth. Wash the parsley, potatoes, dry it, reserve some whole leaves for decorating and chop the rest. Grate the Parmesan cheese.
2. Poach the garlic and onion. Peel and clean the garlic and onion, and chop them. In a casserole with olive oil, beat them for about 5 minutes or so over low heat.
3. Skip the mushrooms. Meanwhile, clean the mushrooms. Leave a few whole pieces for decoration and the rest of the pieces in small pieces. Add them all to the casserole and sauté everything around five more minutes.
4. Make the risotto. Pour the glass of white wine and the broth, and cook for 15 minutes, stirring frequently, and adding broth as the rice absorbs it.
5. Complete the risotto. After the indicated time, add the cheese, parsley, salt and pepper to taste, and the rest of the broth and cook for three more minutes, stirring vigorously. Let stand 2 minutes, and serve.

Nutrition: calories 111, fat 2g, fiber 0g, carbs 8g, protein 6g

Day 30

Breakfast:
Smoked Sausage with Special Dip

Preparation Time: 10 minutes
Cooking Time: 15 minutes
Servings: 4
Ingredients:

- 16 oz. smoked sausage
- 2 tbsp. Dijon mustard
- 3 tbsp. horseradish
- 2 cups shredded cheddar cheese
- ½ cup mayonnaise
- 1 cup green onions (chopped)

Directions:

1. In a large, non-stick skillet, fry the sausages for about 3 to 5 minutes or until they change color.
2. Once cooked, remove excess oil using a paper towel.
3. Mix the rest of the ingredients in a bowl and heat in the microwave for about 60 seconds.
4. Stir the mixture until smooth. If lumps are still present, heat again if necessary.
5. Serve and enjoy!

Nutrition: calories 535, fat 34g, fiber 2g, carbs 18g, protein 33g

Snack
Warm Chicken Salad
Preparation Time: 10 minutes
Cooking Time: 40 minutes
Servings: 4
Ingredients:
- 250 g Chicken breast
- ½ head Lettuce
- ½ head cabbage
- 1 cucumber
- 1 onion (chopped)
- 5 cherry tomatoes
- 1 avocado
- ½ cup egg mayonnaise
- 2 tbsp. balsamic vinegar
- Ground coriander (for seasoning)
- Salt (for seasoning)
- Black pepper (for seasoning)
- 2 tbsp. Olive oil

Directions:
For the chicken:
1. Take the chicken breast and coat it in a mixture of salt, pepper and coriander.
2. Once coated, take a frying pan and heat the olive oil over medium heat.
3. Fry the chicken until crisp and golden brown.
4. Serve and enjoy.

Nutrition: calories 430, fat 8g, fiber 2g, carbs 8g, protein 19g

Lunch:
Low-carb Slow-cooked Pizza

Preparation time: 10 Minutes
Cooking time: 35 Minutes
Serving: 2
Ingredients:
- ¾ lb. ground beef, cooked
- 3/4 lb. Italian sausage, cooked
- 3 cups mozzarella cheese, shredded
- 16 slices low-carb pepperoni
- 1 15 oz. can pizza sauce
- 1 Onions, chopped
- 3 cups fresh spinach
- Any favorite topping like olives, mushrooms or herbs

Directions:
1. Slice the sausage, chop the onions and combine them with the pizza sauce. Divide the mixture in half and put one half into the slow cooker
2. Layer half of the fresh spinach on top of the sauce mixture
3. Layer half of the pepperoni and the remaining toppings on top.
4. Top with half of the cheese.
5. Repeat layers and cook for 6 hours. Let cool slightly before cutting and serving.

Nutrition: calories 186, fat 11g, fiber 2g, carbs 5g, protein 612g

Dinner:
Bone-in Za'atar Chops

Preparation time: 10 minutes
Cooking Time: 10 minutes
Serving: 2
Ingredients:
- 8 pork loin chops, bone-in
- 1 tbsp. Za'atar
- 3 garlic cloves, crushed
- 1 tsp. avocado oil
- 2 tbsp. lemon juice
- 1 1/4 tsp. salt
- Black pepper, to taste

Directions:
1. Rub the pork chops with oil, za'atar, salt, lemon juice, garlic, and black pepper.
2. Place these chops in the Air fryer basket.
3. Press "Power Button" of Air Fry Oven and turn the dial to select the "Air Fry" mode.
4. Press the Time button and again turn the dial to set the cooking time to 10 minutes.
5. Now push the Temp button and rotate the dial to set the temperature at 400°F.
6. Once preheated, place the air fryer basket in the oven and close its lid.
7. Flip the chops when cooked halfway through then resume cooking.
8. Serve warm.

Nutrition: calories 391, fat 8g, fiber 2g, carbs 23g, protein 26g

Day 31

Breakfast:
Pear and Pecan Salad

Preparation Time: *10 minutes*
Cooking Time: *30 minutes*
Servings: *6*
Ingredients:
- ½ cup Gouda cheese
- ½ cup pecans (halved)
- 1 tbsp. unsalted butter
- 3 tbsp. walnut oil
- 1 medium sized pear (sliced into wedges)
- 1/8 tsp. curry powder
- ¾ tsp. salt
- ¼ tsp. freshly ground black pepper
- ¾ cup wine vinegar
- 2 tsps. sucralose sweetener
- 10 cups salad leaves (lightly packed)
- 1/8 tsp. red pepper
- ¾ cup white wine vinegar

Direction
1. In a medium sized non-stick skillet, melt the butter over medium heat.
2. Add in the pecans, 1 tsp. of the sucralose, salt and cayenne pepper and vinegar
3. Add the rest of the ingredients
4. Stir the mixture using a wooden spoon for about 4-5 minutes Utes, or until the pecans are toasted evenly.
5. Make sure that the nuts are coated well with the spices.
6. Set aside in a small bowl to cool.

Nutrition: calories 224, fat 13g, fiber 2g, carbs 8g, protein 61g

Snack
Italian Squash Pie
Preparation Time: 10 minutes
Cooking Time: 45 minutes
Servings: 8
Ingredients:
- 4 tbsp. butter
- 1 ½ lbs. yellow, summer squash (sliced thinly)
- 1 small onion (chopped finely)
- 1 clove garlic (minced)
- ½ tsp. salt
- 2 tsp. Italian seasoning
- ¼ cup parsley (chopped)
- 1 cup Monterey jack cheese (shredded)
- 2 eggs
- ¼ cup heavy cream
- 2 tsp. Dijon mustard

Directions:
1. Preheat the oven to 375°F.
2. In a large saucepan sauté in butter the following: squash, onion, and garlic.
3. Cook until tender and lightly browned.
4. Sprinkle in the seasoning while cooking.
5. In a greased 10-inch quiche pan, place the squash mixture.
6. Add in cheese and parsley.
7. In a small bowl, whisk the eggs and cream together.
8. Add in the mustard and blend well.
9. Pour in this mixture over the quiche pan and fold in gently.
10. Bake in the oven for about 25 minutes.
11. Once done, allow the pan to cool on a rack before cutting the pie.

Nutrition: calories 176, fat 8g, fiber 2g, carbs 7g, protein 23g

Lunch:

Cajun Tofu

Preparation time: 10 Minutes
Cooking time: 20 Minutes
Serving: 2
Ingredients:

- 6 oz. firm tofu, sliced into cubes
- 1 tsp. olive oil
- 1 tbsp. Cajun rub

Directions:

1. Pat the tofu dry using a paper towel.
2. Season with the Cajun rub.
3. Pour the olive oil into the Instant Pot.
4. Set it to sauté.
5. Fry until golden.

Nutrition: calories 76, fat 6g, fiber 2g, carbs 5g, protein 7g

Dinner:
Quinoa confetti

Preparation time: 10 Minutes

Cooking time: 35 Minutes

Serving: 2

Ingredients:

- 1 1/2 cups vegetable stock (low sodium) or water
- 1 cup well-washed and drained quinoa
- 1/2 tsp. salt
- 1/2 tsp. black pepper
- 1 cup mixed frozen vegetables (carrots, peas, corn, etc.)

Directions:

1. Add the vegetable stock or water in a medium saucepan over medium heat and bring everything to a boil.
2. Add quinoa, salt, and pepper, reduce to low heat and cover the pan with a lid. Cook until the liquid evaporate and the quinoa is soft for about 15 minutes. Remove the lid, pour in the vegetables and move it with a fork. Cover again so that the vegetables are cooked with the steam of quinoa.

Nutrition: calories 286, fat 6g, fiber 2g, carbs 5g, protein 7g

ΧΗΑΠΤΕΡ 9:

Atkins Diet and Intermittent Fasting

Atkins diet

The Atkins diet allows protein and fat. The human body cannot store the protein, and therefore, excess amounts are eliminated. The fat, in turn, cannot be processed without the carbohydrates.

The Atkins diet is based on the assumption that carbohydrates are needed to metabolize fats.

If these are no longer supplied, the fat absorbed by the food can no longer be processed and excreted. Also, quitting consumption of carbohydrates leads to a change in metabolism. Carbohydrates are absorbed quickly into the blood and quickly increase blood sugar levels. By eliminating carbohydrates, the blood sugar level remains constantly low. A low blood sugar level, in turn, stimulates fat burning, which in spite of high fat intake in the Atkins diet, leads to the breakdown of the stored fat reserves. This describes the state of ketosis desired in the Atkins diet.

It is a perfect diet for fast-paced and busy lifestyles. You will lose weight without any exercise.

Your body will be doing all the work for you. If you do not follow the Atkins Diet strictly, you will not lose weight. There is no calorie counting nor strict exercise regimens in the Atkins diet. Committing to the Atkins Diet does not take time out of your daily routine; rather, it is a change in your way of eating.

All that is asked of you in this diet is to stick to the diet plan as strictly as possible. Eventually, the types of foods that you can eat and in what quantities will become second nature and you will automatically know what to do.

Some people find it fairly easy to cut back on carbs and have great success without any problems on the Atkins diet. Other people, however, have more difficulty switching to the Atkins diet. It can be a surprise to go from eating much of your caloric intake in carbs to moving to a very low-carb diet, but, with the following keys to success, you will be able to transition more smoothly.

What many people are not aware of is the fact that the body can also utilize fat for energy. When there is no easily accessible sugar (as found in carbohydrates) to break down for energy, the body will turn to fat for the needed energy. Breaking down fat will release stored sugars that can then be used for fuel. Breaking down the fat in your body for sugar will then result in weight loss as these fat cells are destroyed. This process of burning fat for energy is called "lipolysis." When lipolysis takes place and the existing stores of fat are burned, the body then releases something called "ketones." By eating a diet that is low in carbohydrates, you are forcing your body into lipolysis. This process can be maintained by eating a diet that is high in fats as it tricks your body into thinking that the fats that you are consuming are part of the natural process of lipolysis.

Studies have shown that people who have lost weight decrease their risk of colon and breast cancer, even in survivors who are at risk of recurrence.

If you have diabetes, going low-carb can be good for you. Many different studies have verified that following a low-carb diet, such as the Atkins Diet can decrease the symptoms of diabetes, improve the problem of insulin resistance, and can help with different metabolic disorders. Low-carb diets were also shown to improve the problem of daytime sleepiness in people who suffer from narcolepsy, a disorder where people uncontrollably fall asleep during the day. As you can see, there are many benefits to following the Atkins Diet. If you suffer from any of these diseases, you could see some significant improvements in a variety of medical disorders in addition to losing weight by following a low-carb eating plan.

Intermittent Fasting

There has been a lot of buzz around intermittent fasting that it can become difficult to tell it apart from other weight loss diet fads. Intermittent fasting isn't a product; rather, it involves a lifestyle change that requires you to review the times you eat so that you're alternating between periods of fasting and eating. Generally, you'll have more hours of fasting compared to your hours of eating. As a result, you'll experience fat loss because your body is burning and using the stored fat for its fuel when you're in the fasted state. You don't have to make any drastic changes to your lifestyle like the foods you eat or even take chemicals or supplements to speed up the manifestation of the benefits.

Unlike many diet fads you may have tried before, intermittent fasting continues to deliver results for many people. The secret to succeeding with this method of health and wellness is to begin gradually, listen to your body, and make adjustments where necessary. Interestingly, intermittent fasting isn't based on restricting calories. It also doesn't dictate the kind of food you should eat. Instead, you eat your foods normally, so you don't have to give up some foods. Calorie restriction takes place naturally since you have a shorter feeding window. This pattern of feeding helps you to live a healthy lifestyle. This is unlike most diets that leave you with the temptation to eat more than you did before, hence resulting in weight gain. Intermittent fasting is easy to follow through because all you need to do is pay attention to when you eat. Moreover, you're free to take fluids during your fasting window, so that eliminate the possibility of binge eating during the feasting window. There are various disadvantages of eating continually, particularly those foods containing free radicals. Thus, taking a rest from eating allows your body to rest from digestive processes. If you're not sure about embracing intermittent fasting for weight loss, here are some reasons you should consider this pattern of eating over dieting:

It's convenient.

Diets can be demanding. In fact, one of the main reasons why most people abandon diets is because of the inability to follow through. Meeting various life's daily demands that require your attention alongside dieting can be a huge challenge. Intermittent fasting frees up the time you'd have spent preparing meals because you're essentially skipping a number of meals in a day. This means you have fewer instances of decision making. Moreover, you don't have to worry about moving away from your usual food choices as long as you're emphasizing on eating healthy whole foods. This is contrary to most diets that happen to be complex and expensive altogether, yet they don't produce the desired results.

Fasting strengthens your will power.

Your intermittent fasting success is dependent on self-discipline. Intermittent fasting calls for you to be able to resist food even when you're tempted to eat. In the long run, this strengthens your capacity to stay focused and ignore distractions, not just with food but other areas of your life as well. This eventually improves your ability to stay focused and focus on achieving your goals. When you fast, you become more alert and focused; thus, you can ignore any distractions that may come your way to achieve a set goal.

It's a great way to transition into a healthy lifestyle.

Let's face it, most people find it difficult to stick to eating unprocessed foods even though they desire to. After all, processed foods are easily accessible, and they taste better. Intermittent fasting is a great way towards a lifestyle change because while it doesn't explicitly spell out the foods you should eat or avoid, you'll have better results when you include healthy foods in your meals. When your body adjusts to a shorter feeding window, you eliminate the temptation of eating junk food when hunger strikes.

It saves you money and time.

Diets are generally expensive because you have to shop for specific food items and follow the menu to the letter in order to get certain results. This is in addition to the time you'll spend in meal preparation throughout the day. This is usually draining and a burden to your lifestyle. By fasting, you get to save resources and time.

You can incorporate it into your social gatherings.

When you're on a diet, it's unlikely that you'll be able to fit into social gatherings without having to worry about what you'll eat. With intermittent fasting, you can work out your schedule in a way that your feeding window falls within the time when you're most likely to attend social gathers. This way, you won't have to miss out on special occasions or even go out with friends.

Heightened hunger awareness.

Feelings of thirst and hunger are processed by the same part of your brain. As such, it's common to find that you're eating after every two hours because of other reasons that are manifesting as hunger. This could be feelings of boredom, stress, sadness, or happiness. Did you know that the smell of food can make you assume you're hungry? When you fast, your hunger awareness is heightened so that you actually know what it feels like to be hungry and can differentiate between the feel of hunger that is linked to other factors.

Improved quality of sleep.

Most people who adopt the intermittent fasting lifestyle are motivated by the desire to shed excess weight. This might also be a case for you. What you don't know is that with it comes other benefits like better sleep. The reason for this is simple. When you're fasting, your body will mostly digest food before you go to bed. When your fat and insulin levels are kept in check, the quality of your sleep improves.

Conclusion

Keep in mind, it will get easier over time because your strategies to keep the pounds off will eventually become like second nature to you and require little to no effort on your part.

As you have discovered throughout this entire book, the Atkins diet is certainly an option for your body that will make a real difference. The Atkins diet will be easy for you to handle when you understand the proper foods to have.

This diet works with an extensive variety of great foods that are easy for you to consume. They will certainly work wonders for your body as they will help you burn off fat.

It is true, the journey won't be easy, but it is do-able. All you need is motivation and willpower to implement the diet; once you start to see the changes you're looking for, you will find motivation all on your own. Soon you'll fulfill your goals and look your best with your healthy body!

Make a conscious decision to maintain your health and understand what your body does with what you give it, and apply what you've learned! This guidebook comes with a whole passel of recipes and snack ideas. Amaze your friends with your cooking: in their brainwashed minds, perhaps, they'll think your high-fat creams and butter usages are simply crazy. But you will understand the science behind the cream you pour on your pork medallions. You'll understand why you can eat an entire slice of cheesecake and still say you're on a diet.

Good luck in your effort to complete the Atkins diet. You will certainly be proud of yourself when you see just how better and healthier your body is when you use this diet to your advantage.

Thank you.

CPSIA information can be obtained
at www.ICGtesting.com
Printed in the USA
LVHW050322210121
676966LV00009B/498

9 781801 544436